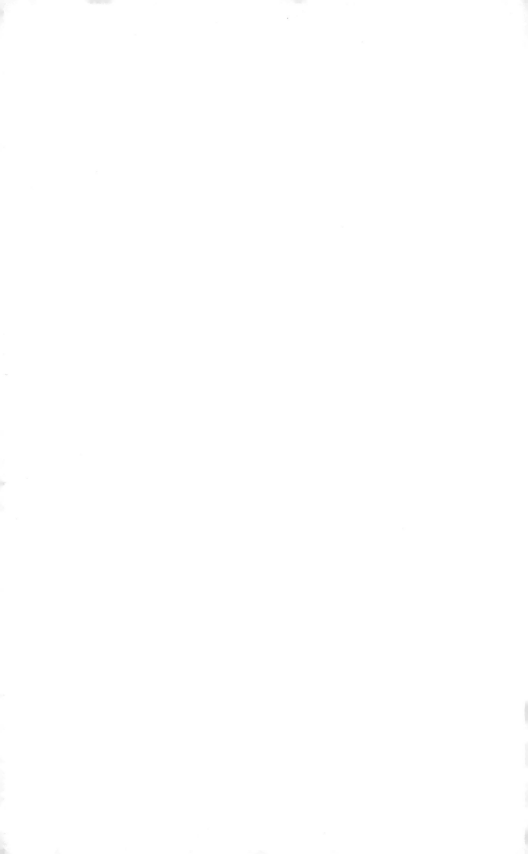

A LIFE EVERLASTING

A LIFE EVERLASTING

*The Extraordinary Story of One
Boy's Gift to Medical Science*

SARAH GRAY

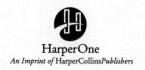

HarperOne
An Imprint of HarperCollinsPublishers

HarperOne

Some of the names in this book have been changed. This book contains a retelling of the story to the best of my ability. There are some parts I remember better than others.

HarperCollins books may be purchased for educational, business, or sales promotional use. For information, please email the Special Markets Department at SPsales@harpercollins.com.

FIRST EDITION

Designed by Joan Olson

Library of Congress Cataloging-in-Publication Data

Names: Gray, Sarah, 1973- author.
Title: A life everlasting: the extraordinary story of one boy's gift to medical science / Sarah Gray.
Description: New York, NY: HarperOne, 2016.
Identifiers: LCCN 2016011725 | ISBN 9780062438225 (hardback) | ISBN 9780062563484 (audio) | ISBN 9780062438249 (ebook)
Subjects: LCSH: Gray, Sarah, 1973—Health. | Gray, Thomas Ethan—Health. | Anencephaly—Patients—Biography. | Mother and infant—United States—Biography. | Organ donors—Biography. | BISAC: BIOGRAPHY & AUTOBIOGRAPHY / Personal Memoirs. | BIOGRAPHY & AUTOBIOGRAPHY / Medical. | MEDICAL / Research.
Classification: LCC QM695.B7 G73 2016 | DDC 362.196830092 [B] — dc23 LC record available at https://lccn.loc.gov/2016011725

16 17 18 19 20   RRD(H)   10 9 8 7 6 5 4 3 2 1

*For everyone who has ever donated
their body for the benefit of others,
and for their families.
For the trusted stewards of these precious gifts.
For the researchers who help those they will never meet.*

And for Thomas.

The child we had, but never had,
And yet we'll have forever.
—from "To the Child in My Heart"
(author unknown)

CONTENTS

PROLOGUE

I decided to give it one last shot. If I was willing to make one of the weirdest calls of my life, maybe something would happen.

I paced the skywalk of the Hynes Convention Center as I imagined how the call might go: I would explain the whole story, and they would tell me it violated some confidentiality thing. Or that it wasn't allowed. Or it wasn't within policy. But I thought, *I have a personal connection to this place. I gave them something they needed. I'm sure they have wondered, at some point, where the donations came from. I'm just going to call. I will feel awkward. Maybe they'll feel awkward, too. If I could just get past the part of talking about the death of a child to a complete stranger over the phone, something powerful might happen. I have to at least try.*

My heart raced as I clicked "Dial," and I gripped the phone hard.

Here goes. I am doing this.

"Hello," a woman's voice said.

Adrenaline shot through me. I tried to play it cool: Shucks, I'm just a regular old girl next door looking for her deceased child's cornea researcher. Just like everybody else.

"Hi, my name is Sarah Gray. I have a kind of unusual request."

CHAPTER ONE

It Wasn't Supposed to Happen Like This

2009

I found out I'm pregnant on August 9, right after our vacation
to Scotland and Italy. Found out it's twins on September 4.
What a shock! We have ultrasound photos and look forward
to getting more in 2 weeks. Praying everything is OK.
—Sarah's journal

Oh—and there *is* another heartbeat," he said.

Dr. John Maddox, my OB-GYN, pointed at a flickering white blob on the plasma screen mounted on the wall.

"Ha, ha. Very funny."

"It's twins," he said, ignoring me. "See here?"

I looked at the screen at what appeared to be two pixelated white kidney beans. Ross and I gave each other a look. I smiled. Ross looked worried.

We had been trying to have a baby for two years, and at thirty-five years old I had been starting to worry it would never happen. We were thrilled to see the positive home pregnancy test I'd taken a couple of weeks earlier, but we never expected twins. We didn't think of ourselves as twins people, whatever that means. "Can you tell if they are fraternal or identical?"

Was this really happening?

"Identical."

I looked over at Ross. His expression seemed to say, *This is more than I bargained for.*

"Can you tell the sex?" I asked.

"It's too early now," Dr. Maddox said, "but we will be able to tell in another four weeks."

The doctor looked at my chart for a few moments.

"Since you're over thirty-five, you might be interested in getting a first-trimester screening—it's up to you." He scribbled something down on his prescription pad, tore it off, and handed it to me. It was a referral to the Genetics & IVF Institute in Fairfax, Virginia. "You can schedule it in the next three or four weeks. They check for genetic defects." Apparently, I was officially an MOAA—a mother of advanced age. (I couldn't help but think of the ROUS—the rodents of unusual size from *The Princess Bride*.)

As we left the office, Ross and I stopped and turned to each other. At eight weeks, it was too early to make any general announcements to family and friends, but we agreed to share this exciting development with the two people who would be the most thrilled: "We've gotta call our moms."

On the way to the car I had a pregnancy craving, so we stopped by a nearby Wendy's for some chicken nuggets and an M&M Twisted Frosty while we called our mothers.

"How are we going to afford this?" Ross asked a bit later, when the excitement had died down. We already knew we'd have to struggle to afford one child, let alone two. "And where are we going to put two cribs?" We lived in a two-bedroom, one-bathroom condo in Northwest Washington, DC. What could have been a cozy home for a family of three suddenly seemed too small for a family of four. It was a second-floor walk-up—no elevator—so we were going to be carrying two children, plus a twin stroller, up and down the stairs every time we went out. It was often difficult to find a parking spot on our street, too, so we regularly ended up parking several blocks away.

Nevertheless, we spent the next few weeks getting used to the idea. We called a real-estate agent to talk about putting our place on the market and looking for a bigger house out in the suburbs.

And we decided to have the first-trimester screening. If more information was available, we would rather know it than not.

"What would we do if there is problem?" Ross asked one evening as he sat at the computer.

The last thing either of us wanted to do was terminate the pregnancy that we had been so longing for. It was too stressful to think about; and anyway, it was hypothetical. Why give ourselves heartache over a choice we might never need to make?

"I don't know," I said. "Let's cross that bridge when we come to it. And hopefully, we will never come to it."

Ross agreed.

We scoured the web in the days before the screening to bone up on the terms we might hear. We wanted to be able to ask the right questions during our appointment. We learned that the ultrasound technician would look for the presence of the fetal nasal bone and measure the nuchal translucency—the size of the clear space in the tissue at the back of a baby's neck. We knew that a measurement of 2.5 millimeters or more in the nuchal fold could indicate Down syndrome. Since I was a thirty-five-year-old MOAA, I had a higher risk of having a child with Down syndrome. It's the most common birth defect in the United States, appearing in approximately one in seven hundred births every year. If we were going to hear any bad news at this appointment, I thought it would be that both twins had Down syndrome, since they were identical.

On the day of the test, per the doctor's request I arrived with a full bladder, which helps push everything into the right place and makes the babies easier to see on the sonogram.

During the sonogram, we could see everything the tech was looking at on a plasma screen mounted on the wall. I recognized the babies' noses, cheeks, arms, legs, and toes. The tech hit the print button a few times, and curling white paper hummed out of the machine. After one first-trimester miscarriage, two years of trying to conceive, and buying numerous adorable baby gifts for friends, finally it was our turn. I had been looking forward to this moment my entire life.

"So does everything look okay?" I asked.

"I'm not allowed to interpret results," the tech said. "The doctor will do that when he comes in. Try to empty your bladder halfway. The restroom is the first door to the left—and when you come back, the doctor will see you."

When she left the room, Ross whispered, "I saw her do the nuchal fold test. The measurement was normal." According to Ross's Internet expertise, we were in the clear.

"I counted the fingers on Baby B," I confided. "Five fingers on the hand I saw."

It was hard to guess how much pee was half the pee in my bladder, but I did my best. After I came back from the bathroom, a gray-haired man in a white coat opened the door and introduced himself as Dr. Stern.

Dr. Stern sat on the stool in front of the sonogram machine and pushed the wand across my belly for about five minutes from a variety of angles. He didn't seem to be getting the angle he needed. He looked concerned.

Then, he put down the wand.

He said, "I'm sorry to tell you that Baby A has a lethal birth defect."

Wait.

What?

Did he just say that?

It felt like the floor had dropped out of the room. The babies we had seen on the screen looked fine: legs kicking, round little butts, cute button noses. The nuchal fold was fine.

"It's called 'acrania,' which means the baby's skull was not fully formed in the early stages of development."

"How do you know that? What do you see?" I asked.

"See how Baby B's skull is round?" Dr. Stern pointed at the frozen image on the screen. "This skull developed properly. Now, look at Baby A's skull. See these bumps? That is exposed brain matter. That shows us that the skull did not close. Also, see how Baby A's amniotic sac is cloudy? The brain matter has disintegrated into the fluid. Baby B's amniotic fluid is clear."

Dr. Stern paused.

"Do you have any questions for me?"

I took a deep breath and collected myself. "What causes this?" I asked, my mind racing to all the things I might have done that could cause birth defects.

When I first stopped taking birth-control pills a couple of years earlier, I had expected and hoped to get pregnant quickly. I was diligent about following medical recommendations, common wisdom, and even old wives' tales about what to do for a healthy pregnancy. I took prenatal vitamins, cut back on alcohol, switched to decaffeinated coffee, and avoided hot tubs, sushi, soft cheese, and lunch meat.

Eventually, however, after months of negative pregnancy tests, I slowly reincorporated caffeinated coffee and wine into my routine.

Then I remembered our vacation in Scotland and Italy two months earlier. In Scotland, I had been caught in a cold downpour without an umbrella and was chilled to the bone, so I took advantage of the hotel's hot tub and sauna to warm up. I knew that hot tubs often had warning signs for pregnant women, so even though I didn't know at the time that I was pregnant, I was careful not to stay in either very long—maybe five minutes in the bath-temperature hot tub and another ten minutes in the sauna.

I'd compounded the situation in Italy when we toured Pompeii on a hot, dry August day. The temperature hit well into the nineties, and because of the devastating eruption of Mount Vesuvius in AD 79, the site harbors little in the way of shade trees. Walking around the temples of Apollo and Jupiter, the Forum, and the House of the Faun, I was desperate enough that I drank out of the dilapidated brass water fountains; the water was hot. Maybe I was overheated that day?

Later on in the trip, we took a ferry from Naples to the island of Ischia and visited the Negombo thermal spa resort. There were signs about not entering the spa if you were pregnant. For two years, I had been in a state of possibly being pregnant. Most of the time, I wasn't. I decided to go in the cool and warm thermal pools but only dip my feet in the hot ones.

Now I wondered, was it the heat?

Or could it be alcohol? There was the champagne at Ross's sister's wedding. And there was the pub crawl with friends in Edinburgh. We won third place in a pub quiz, and the prize was a round of neon-colored test-tube shots. In Italy, we had enjoyed the local wine and drunk the limoncello we made from the lemons in my friend's yard.

"It's a neural tube defect," Dr. Stern said. "Low levels of folic acid in the diet can be a cause."

Folic-acid deficiency? That's for rookies. Everyone knows to take folic acid. Doctors had been recommending it as a standard supplement since 1992. Even breakfast cereals and bread are fortified with folic acid. Folic acid I definitely did right. But even if I had been folic-acid deficient . . . why did only one twin have acrania? "I have been taking a prenatal vitamin almost every day for about two years now," I said. "And I eat food that probably has even more folic acid in it. Could it be something else?"

Dr. Stern looked uncomfortable, as though he had already exhausted his knowledge of this topic.

"Are either of you from Belfast? There has been a higher concentration of incidences there."

My mind was reeling. I had not read this on Babycenter. com. What did being from Belfast have to do with it? I had never been to Belfast, but I imagined the citizens as 100 percent having brains.

My cell phone rang in my purse. I fumbled to turn it off without taking it out.

"I have Irish ancestors, but none from Belfast. And that was two hundred years ago. Ross was born in Scotland—"

"Scotland is *not* Ireland!" Ross interrupted, indignant.

"I used a sauna before I knew I was pregnant. Or could it be something I ate or drank? Like sushi or wine?"

I pictured myself on a bus poster with a serious face and the words *I ate a rainbow roll and it killed my baby. Don't take chances.*

"There have not been a lot of studies, and the ones that I have read are not conclusive."

We were obviously asking for information that he didn't have. I felt sorry for Dr. Stern: he had to tell us the news with barely any knowledge of the cause.

"Have you ever seen a baby like this before? How often do you see this? Like, once a year?"

"Yes, about once a year."

Okay, so this is pretty rare.

"What do the babies look like?"

He looked at the wall a moment before answering. He took a deep breath.

"The skull stops near the eyebrows." He lifted his hand to his brow line, in a kind of salute. "The brain is exposed at the top." He paused and lowered his voice. "Sometimes it looks like the baby is wearing a mask."

I thought I knew about all the basic birth defects. This one sounded too bizarre and terrible to be true. How would we feel when we saw this baby? Would we be scared?

"Is Baby B okay?" I asked.

"Baby B appears to be fine. I don't see anything of any concern at this point, although things could change. But the nuchal fold looks good, so I'm not concerned about Down syndrome."

Ross and I nodded.

"Is there anything we can do?" I asked.

"You have a few options. You can terminate this pregnancy and try again. Or you could carry both twins to term. Baby B would be born healthy, and Baby A will be stillborn or die within a few minutes or hours."

"What will be the actual cause of death?"

"The part of the brain that regulates heartbeat and body temperature is missing. So the trauma of being born can cause the heart to stop. Right now, your heartbeat is keeping both babies alive. Once the umbilical cord is cut, Baby A will begin to die."

Giving birth to one healthy baby and one dead baby seemed like a sick joke.

What kind of God takes away a child's brain? What kind of sicko makes a mother gestate a baby for nine months only to have the baby die at the moment of birth? Who came up with this? And are they ashamed of themselves?

And why me? Why my child? Is it something I did? Don't I follow the rules? God, if you are trying to teach me a lesson, and you are merciful and forgiving like I thought you were, why didn't you just send me a message in a dream? There are so many other ways of communicating. Killing a baby is not fighting fair. Take this up with me, not them.

"Should we look into selective termination?" I asked.

I remembered the phrase from watching the TLC reality show *John & Kate Plus 8.* John and Kate already had twins when they decided to try for another child. A round of in vitro fertilization (IVF) produced not one more, not two, but seven embryos (though one eventually disappeared). Before the treatment, the couple had expressly hoped for just one more child but had also stated that they would not selectively terminate; the procedure is used if there is a defect or to protect the health of the other babies and the mom. And the phrase, though horribly clinical, had stuck in my head, especially when their family of four had become a famous family of ten.

"You won't be able to do that, because these are identical twins and they share a placenta. What happens to one will affect the other." Dr. Stern went on to explain that my babies were mono-di, or monochorionic diamniotic, twins, which meant that each had its own amniotic sac, but they shared a placenta.

Mono-di twins begin as a single sperm and a single egg. Together these form a zygote, which splits into two somewhere between four and eight days later and creates what we know as identical twins. I sometimes think about those four to eight days. When exactly did the split happen? What was I doing when it did?

And then all of a sudden those what-ifs receded and I realized how lucky I was that we would possibly still have one healthy child. It was all we had hoped for in the first place. I had gone into this exam assuming that if we had a child with a birth defect, we would be faced with the choice we didn't want in the first place—the choice to terminate. But because that child had a healthy identical twin, we would not even have that terrible option.

My mind jumped ahead to the delivery. I had always hoped to become a mother. While I was scared of the pain of delivery, I looked forward to finding out for myself what it feels like to bring a new life into the world. I assumed that I would be excited and happy on the day my child was born. It started to dawn on me that it would be the opposite. I might actually dread the moment my children were born.

And right there, before I'd even left the sonogram room, I found myself starting to recalculate. A fuzzy plan started to form, which I hoped would lead to a way to cope with this new reality.

Perhaps the way to think of it was that we were having one child, which is what Ross and I had originally planned for. Baby B was the baby we always wanted. Maybe I could think of Baby A as a necessary complication. I didn't picture myself holding this baby or giving it a name. Since Dr. Stern didn't have much experience with this birth defect, maybe that was true of the medical community as a whole. I wondered if studying the baby's body might be helpful to scientists.

"Maybe after the birth, we could donate the baby's body to science?" I asked. I imagined birthing a healthy Baby B while nurses whisked away Baby A. I still hoped that this pregnancy could be a happy one. And perhaps I could find a hidden reason for this terrible situation.

Dr. Stern hesitated. "I am not sure how that would work."

"I would want to give the baby a proper burial," Ross said. He had been sitting in silence the entire time, but now he looked a little offended.

It was clear that the doctor's job was done. My questions were multiplying in my head, but I had already asked more than Dr. Stern could answer. We would need other experts now: a genetic counselor, a high-risk-pregnancy ob-gyn.

A funeral director.

There was one last thing I had to ask.

"Can I keep the sonogram pictures you showed us?"

"Are you sure you want these? Some people don't like to keep them."

These were the most important pictures that had ever been taken of anything in our lives. I wanted to keep them, so I did.

Dr. Stern offered to put us in touch with a genetic counselor, then left Ross and me alone.

Ross and I gripped each other in a hard hug and said nothing for a minute. I could feel his heart pounding in his chest.

It had been only a few days earlier that the real-estate agent had stopped by to talk about painting our condo to get it ready to sell because we'd need more room. . . . My brother Mark had emailed me the name of the paint color that I liked in his living room: Sandstone Cove. None of that would be necessary anymore. We went from expecting one baby, to twins, to a healthy child and a dead one.

My cell phone vibrated in my purse again. I reached in to see who was calling. It was someone from work. I hit "Ignore" and swore to myself that I would never again call someone who said he or she was going to a doctor's appointment.

Ross finally said, "I can't hold the baby while it dies. I can't. I know I'm not going to be able to do that."

"Let's take our time and talk about it. Can you take the rest of the day off? This is a legitimate family emergency."

And to think that I thought sonograms were supposed to be fun. This one had been terrible.

We hurried out of the office, past the modern decor and large fish tanks in the lobby, keeping our eyes firmly to the floor. I didn't want to make eye contact with any staff members, in case they knew. *That's them, the couple with the freak diagnosis.*

Ross and I got in our separate cars—we had each come from our jobs—to email our bosses that we wouldn't be returning to work. Then I called my mom, a registered nurse. She knew what was at stake.

"How'd it go?" my mom asked me when I reached her.

"It's not good."

I knew her heart was breaking, too. She was just as excited as we were—probably even more so. These were her grandchildren. . . .

When I got home half an hour later I parked in front of our building and called my colleague Susan, who works at the Pentagon, back to deal with the work issue that she'd been calling about. I had been working for six years in marketing at NISH, formerly National Industries for the Severely Handicapped. NISH supports a federal government program that helps secure contracts for nonprofit agencies that employ people with disabilities. In my communications and marketing role, I founded and managed a speakers' bureau and helped people with disabilities, mostly wounded veterans, become advocates for hiring people with disabilities. Susan was a client but also a mentor and confidante. Normally, I would have had a focused approach to whatever was going on at work, but I felt like I was an astronaut floating in outer space.

I told Susan what had happened.

"Oh my gosh, Sarah. Oh my gosh." Susan took a breath. "I am so happy for you, but so sad, too. I will be praying for you."

When I walked in the door of our condo, Ross was talking on the phone to his mother in Scotland while looking up *acrania* on the Internet. I collapsed onto the bed.

Ross hung up the phone and came over to lie down next to me.

"What did you learn?" I asked.

"It will progress into something called anencephaly." This was all so new he wasn't even sure how to pronounce the word. "Without a proper skull, the brain can't develop. . . ."

"That's what my mom said, too. I guess we should go over all the options—everything we can think of—then take our time to make a decision. Let's just talk it out."

Ross nodded. We lay there for a while, alone and together.

Eventually he said, "We could have an abortion and start over."

"Yes, that's one option. The thing I don't like about that is I don't know when or if I will ever get pregnant again. But it's an option."

Ross nodded again.

"Another one is to carry both to term," I said. "We still have one healthy baby. That's all we expected to have anyway. So, technically, we are still getting what we were hoping for all along."

"If we do that, I don't want to send the baby off to a lab. I want Baby A to be laid to rest in a proper grave, a place for Baby B to visit. I want the baby to feel loved."

"Why are you so attached to Baby A?" I asked him. "I thought you were scared of having twins."

He paused.

Then Ross said, "I wanted both."

We said nothing for a while. Then Ross got off of the bed and went into the living room. I heard him pour himself a single malt, which we reserved for special occasions.

It was autumn. The babies were due in the spring.

CHAPTER TWO

Sophie's Choice, Backward at 100 mph

2004

The flight attendant put those little napkins on our tray tables, handed us our wine, and, thirty-five thousand feet above the Atlantic Ocean, my friend Kim and I clinked plastic.

As we drank, we devised a scavenger hunt for our ten-day vacation in England and Scotland. Among the things we planned, we were going to try to get our pictures taken with all the quirky stereotypes we could think of involving British people: someone who worked at a fish-and-chips shop; someone in a kilt; a bag-piper; a woman named Pippa; and a man named Nigel.

A week later, and with just a couple of days left on our itin-erary, we realized we hadn't made much progress. After dinner in Glasgow, we stopped in at a place called O'Neill's Pub, in the Merchant City part of town, for a pint.

"Is your name Nigel?" I asked a tall, dark-haired stranger.

"Naw."

I started thinking it might be a good idea to recruit a local to help us.

"We're doing a scavenger hunt. We need to get a picture taken with someone named Nigel. Do you know anyone here named Nigel?"

"Nigel is an English name," non-Nigel said with a burr. He yelled to a friend, "Paul! You know anyone here called Nigel?"

"Nigel? Naw," he said.

"There's nobody named Nigel in Scotland," the first non-Nigel said. "My name is Ross. That's a better name. A Scottish name. It means 'a headland.' You should get a picture with me instead."

"Ross? Like from the TV show *Friends*?"

"Aye," he nodded.

"Oh . . . sorry, we have the name 'Ross' in America. It's not on the list. Thanks anyway," I said.

Ross introduced Kim and me to his friend Paul, and they asked us about our travels. We told them about our visit to London, Edinburgh, Glasgow Cathedral, and the Necropolis.

"Do you like Scotland?" Paul asked.

"I love it!" I said. "I love the country. I love the people. I love to drink Scotch. I love Scotch tape. Masking tape is for fools."

We soon realized that these men were extremely proud of their homeland and perhaps had been drinking all day. Ross even treated us to his rendition of the Scottish national anthem. "Ohhh flow'r of Scootlannd . . . when will we seee . . . your likes again? Who fought and diiiied for . . . your weeee bit hill and glen—"

"Your what?" I interrupted.

"A glen is a valley."

"What did you say before 'glen'?"

"Hill?"

"Before that . . ."

". . . wee bit?"

"Did you say *wee . . . bit*?" His accent was a challenge. And there was a live band covering Coldplay loudly in the background.

"*Wee* means 'small.'"

"So, a 'wee bit' means a 'small bit,' right, like a small small thing? A small small piece *of what*?"

"It's a wee *bit*. A wee bit . . . in your heart." A noun was still clearly missing, and who knows, perhaps a bunch of other words. He made a pinching motion over his heart and smiled.

Ross was from Stirling (he pronounced it "Stun-lin"), a city halfway between Glasgow and Edinburgh, and he had moved to Glasgow to attend the University of Strathclyde. I told him I was from Falls Church, Virginia, and was getting ready to move to nearby Washington, DC.

"Actually, I have something to celebrate," I said, as we lifted our pints in a toast. "This week, I officially bought my first home. I just faxed the closing documents from our hotel."

It turned out that Paul was actually in town for his grandfather's funeral, and was sleeping over at Ross's flat. I could have talked to Ross longer, but I wondered about Kim. She lived in California; I lived on the East Coast. We hadn't seen each other in at least a year. This trip was as much to catch up with Kim as it was to see the sights. I wasn't there to pick up guys. I said to them, "Nice to meet you," and we excused ourselves to the ladies' room.

"What happened? Didn't you like Ross? He's cute," Kim said.

"Yeah, he is. But I didn't know if you wanted to keep talking to them or what. It's okay," I said. "Let's get another drink."

A few drinks later, Ross and Paul joined us at the bar and we continued our chat. Ross told me that he was a civil engineer and that he designed roads.

"I love roads. I am a big fan," I said, because everyone likes when their work is appreciated. And anyway, where would I be without roads? I probably drove on roads every day of my life. My new house was even on a road! So I said, "If we got married, you could build a road to my new house."

Ross didn't miss a beat; he laughed, then suggested a plan of his own.

"And if we have kids, can I name the girls? Because I already have two names picked out."

"What are they?"

"Jacklyn and Jocelyn. I picked them out a long time ago. You can name the boys."

I didn't really like those names, but this didn't strike me as a binding agreement.

"Okay, it's a deal."

The bartenders yelled for last call, and Paul ordered four whiskeys.

"This is the kindy whiskey ma granddad used ta drink," he said. "Here's a toast him!" he said as he lifted his glass. We raised ours, too.

"Slainte," said Ross, toasting us in Scots Gaelic.

"To granddad," Kim and I said.

Half an hour later we found ourselves in an honest-to-goodness Scottish apartment, or "flat," as they called it.

We had spent almost all of our time on vacation in hotels surrounded by tourists, so it was an easy decision to hang out with some locals. And this being Britain, many of the pubs closed at midnight. It was still relatively early when you're on vacation time. After we left O'Neill's we'd walked two blocks down Bell Street to Ross's place at Parsonage Square, near the High Street train station.

Ross had two roommates, Katy and Web, who were a couple. When we arrived at the flat on Parsonage Square—across from a stone castle–like whiskey warehouse—Web was sitting on the couch with a pint. He had been injured in a rugby game and was trying to drink away the pain. Web spoke in an accent that seemed part Scottish, part leprechaun, though it may have been the combination of painkillers, beer, and, well, pain.

Leaving Web to his sprained whatever, Ross gave me a tour of the flat. I was intrigued by the everyday household things that were different in the United States. He had a breakfast cereal called Shreddies (it seemed like a version of Crispix), and he had Saran Wrap, but he called it Cling Film. The dish soap was called Fairy Liquid.

And then there was the life-size cardboard Ginger Spice in the living room.

Forget Nigel. This was turning into scavenger-hunt gold.

I took a picture of Ross holding Cling Film and washing a dish with Fairy Liquid. Kim and I got photos with the Spice Girl.

There was a future ahead of us, though we didn't know it at the time. All Kim and I knew was that a night in a Scottish pub and flat could lead to some serious headaches the next morning. Oh, and there was a new email address in my contacts. Ross mentioned that a group of his friends were planning to visit New York City over the summer, and we agreed he and I would try to meet up then.

Emails turned to weekly, then daily, phone calls. The plans for a trip to NYC with his friends unraveled, but I offered to show him DC and NYC if he still wanted to visit.

"Are you sure you don't have a boyfriend?" he asked.

"Yeah. Are you sure you don't have a girlfriend?" I asked. "I don't want some Scottish lady with blue paint on her face coming to get me."

And at that, Ross bought a plane ticket to spend a week with me in August. I thought we would get along for a week, but I didn't know for sure. We both secretly arranged another place for him to stay if it wasn't a good match. I decided that no matter how things turned out between us, I would at least show him some cool things in Washington and New York so he would have good memories of the East Coast. Who knew if he would ever be back again?

He arrived at Dulles International, and despite my fears, I recognized him. The next day, he insisted we visit a bar at 7 A.M. to watch the Glasgow Celtic game, and I obliged. We visited the White House, the U.S. Capitol, and the National Mall in Washington, and the Staten Island Ferry, Central Park, and the Empire State Building in New York.

Despite the fact that we spoke the same language, I was surprised by how different our countries and cultures were. He was baffled that on a hot, humid August day when the temperature was over one hundred degrees, there were no patrons who chose to eat outside at the nearby Mexican restaurant.

"It's too hot and humid to be comfortable outside," I explained, pointing out that it wasn't closed; there were customers behind the glass: "I guess they just want to be in the air-conditioning."

He took a moment to collect himself.

"That would never happen in Scotland."

He explained that Scotland gets so few nice, sunny days that Scottish people would never spend time in air-conditioning when they could be in the sun—even if it was miserably uncomfortable—because they didn't know when another sunny day would come along. I remembered our Scottish neighbor from when I was a child who used to sunbathe when the temperature was in the fifties. The neighbors thought she must be freezing, but she would always say it was a lovely day.

I took Ross to a Redskins football game, where he was surprised that the Redskins fans and Panthers fans were not separated. "There is a guy wearing a Panthers jersey *right behind us!*" he whispered, incredulous, as we walked down the stadium ramp after the game.

When I mentioned that I needed to go to the DMV to renew my driver's license, he said, "Oh, where Patty and Selma work?"—referring to Marge Simpson's gravel-voiced sisters on *The Simpsons.* The week was full of moments like these that made me see my own country through the eyes of a tourist.

It was hard to say good-bye when he left, but he said he would come back soon. A month later, I was excitedly driving to the airport to pick him up again.

A transatlantic relationship isn't inexpensive or easy to maintain. After the second trip, we had to a heart-to-heart to figure out if we were both up for this.

"I think we have a future," he said. "Do you?"

I said yes. He said that if it came down to it, he would be willing to move to America. He had lived in California briefly as a child when his father was a visiting professor at Cal State Sacramento. He and his dad had toyed with the notion of making the move permanent, but his mom missed her family back home. By the time we met, Ross had been living in Glasgow for seven years and was ready for a change.

Ross and I ended up dating across the Atlantic for a year and a half. He met my brothers, Mark and Ethan, and my parents. In Scotland, he showed me around different parts of the country and introduced me to a host of Scottish pastimes, including a Celtic football game, a ceilidh (pronounced *kay-lee*), and a gig at the famous music venue King Tut's Wah Wah Hut.

Though Ross grew up in Stirling, his adopted hometown of seven years had been Glasgow. Glasgow is Scotland's largest city and is known for a thriving art and music scene, a unique accent, and colorful locals.

Edinburgh, an hour away, is considered more genteel and beautiful than its sometimes unruly neighbor to the west. We toured the famous castle there, and the Scottish Parliament building, where Ross helped build the first floor when he was still in university. He was working there on September 11, 2001; the building had been evacuated that day, like so many others.

A ceilidh is a traditional Scottish evening of music and danc- ing. The men wore kilts of all different tartans, and the women wore cocktail dresses. Some of the men sneaked pints of vodka under the table, which they mixed with Coke—something I had never seen in America. Everyone seemed to know how to do special dances: "Strip the Willow," the "Dashing White Ser- geant," and the "Gay Gordons." It reminded me of an American square dance. Ross tried to teach me the moves, and no one seemed to care when I did it all wrong. The last song of the evening was "Loch Lomond," and everyone joined in a circle to sing it together. I felt like I had gone two hundred years back in time.

Ross also introduced me to what I would discover is one of his abiding passions: soccer—or, as he calls it, football. He took me to see his favorite team, Celtic, who play at the hallowed Celtic Park. I'd been to sports events in America, but this was a whole other megillah. Fans actually kill each other over these games. Since guns are illegal in Scotland—even the police don't carry them—it's mostly stabbings, a crime that seems almost old-fashioned in America. While games in America can feature kiss-cams, dancing tacos, and prompts to get the fans riled up, games at Celtic Park are noticeably more serious and less orga- nized. The atmosphere has an element of a heated political pro- test about it.

Most of the fans were male and over the age of fifteen. I don't think it's a stretch to say that many of them had had something to drink before they showed up. In terms of audience participation, it seemed to bubble up out of nowhere rather than being led by an emcee or piped-in songs—no *"Charge!"* here. In fact, it seemed to be quite the opposite: no one was trying to get the fans any more riled up than they already were upon arrival. For starters, alcohol is not sold inside the stadium. The opposing team's fans are seated in a sectioned-off part of the stadium, with a cadre of police in stab-proof vests, and sometimes riot shields, escorting them in and out through a separate entrance. Fans have been known to throw batteries, small and undetectable by security, and plastic bags filled with urine at players during a game. Then there were the often-obscene chants about each other, the teams, the referee, and the players, and even bits of political history, not to mention incredible roars when goals were scored. It is fair to say that the harmless, dorky ribbing heard at American games ("Your team sucks!" "Ha, ha—no, your team sucks!") would be tragically misunderstood here. In fact, people have probably been stabbed for less. I think I enjoyed it; I was mostly happy to get out alive.

But it wasn't all dancing and chanting: we had some lovely quiet times, too, times when our love couldn't help but deepen. In Aviemore, a picturesque town two and a half hours north of Glasgow, we strolled around in the shadow of the impressive Cairngorm Mountains. Farther west we visited Glencoe, a beautiful glen in the Scottish Highlands and the site of a legendary clash of Scottish clans.

Ross having introduced me to the salient parts of his country, it was clear that we would take the next step. It was time for us both to head west, to my country, and a new life together. The start of the future had arrived.

Ross moved to Washington, DC, on October 10, 2005, and we got married five days later, paying a justice of the peace thirty dollars to marry us in a gazebo at the Carlyle House, a historic mansion in Alexandria built by John Carlyle, a Scot and one of the founders of the Commonwealth of Virginia.

Then we celebrated as we had begun: we went to Murphy's Pub for a drink.

Four years later, I stopped taking birth-control pills. Then, twins. Then, the sonogram.

After the diagnosis, Ross and I both immersed ourselves in research, digging up everything about acrania and anencephaly we could find on the Internet. (It was a bit of a shock the first time I put those words into Google and discovered there were heavy-metal bands called Acrania and Anencephalic. This told me that our baby's diagnosis was terrifying and repulsive, like something out of a horror movie.)

But I found help as well, from a website called anencephaly. info. Based out of Switzerland, the site was started in November 2000 by a mom named Monika Jaquier, shortly after she lost her infant daughter, Anouk, to the condition. Monika had found such comfort in talking to other families who had been through this experience that she wanted to help others the way she had been helped. This amazing resource—it's published in a number of languages and has been visited by millions of people around the world—is filled with photographs and stories from other moms and dads who had been down the road Ross and I were now traveling. It was a godsend.

One story in particular caught my eye. A woman named Allison Andrews, from Shreveport, Louisiana, also had twins, Sarah and Faith, and Faith had anencephaly. I emailed Allison the day after our diagnosis. She responded the same day, saying she would be happy to talk.

The diagnosis gave us something significant in common. I was grateful that a fellow human being, twelve hundred miles away, was willing to help me just because I would be going through the same thing. She signed off on her email, "Hang in there, girl." My pen pal and I emailed back and forth a number of times, and arranged a phone call two weeks later. Ross listened in to my end of the conversation.

"I am so touched that you emailed me. I have been in your shoes, and I know exactly how you feel," she said.

Hearing those words felt like when a cold shower finally turns warm. My emotions unclenched.

She warned me to expect awkward moments with friends and strangers, and mixed emotions—and she offered practical advice about the labor, and the funeral. We talked about things I would not dare ask anyone else in the world.

"Years before I ever had children, I heard about someone holding a child that died, and I remember thinking, *That's morbid and creepy.* Well, I ate my words!" she said. "Because when it's *your* child, you react however your heart feels. I held Faith for three hours after she passed away, and those hours were precious to me. The hardest part was handing her over to the nurse."

Then she changed the subject, and this one brief exchange changed everything.

"Have you heard about the study at Duke?" Allison asked. She explained that researchers at Duke University were trying to find a cause or a cure for anencephaly. She and her husband, Charles, had contributed cord blood from their twins, along with their own blood, to help advance the study. Not quite realizing how important this would turn out to be, I nevertheless wrote down the words *Duke study.*

As we wrapped up our conversation, I felt a sense of comfort. I was not alone.

"You will never fully heal from it, but it gets better," Allison said. "You will be okay. And call me any time you want to talk."

After we hung up, I felt something I hadn't felt in a while: a smile on my face. I had a new friend.

The Duke Center for Human Genetics (now called the Duke Molecular Physiology Institute) was looking for families who were expecting a newborn diagnosed with anencephaly to participate in a study called "The Hereditary Basis of Neural Tube Defects." The idea was to identify the genes that contribute to the development of the neural tube—the tube-shaped structure in embryos that becomes the brain and spinal cord—with the hopes of developing better preventions and treatments and possibly a cure. Participants were required to speak to a coordinator, complete a medical history, provide a blood sample, and arrange to provide a sample of cord blood from the baby—or, in the case of twins, from both babies. I sent an email to the study contact to see if we might be eligible.

"Are you sure they are identical twins, and not fraternal?" the coordinator, Heidi Cope, asked when we spoke on the phone. She sounded suspicious.

"Yes, that's what my doctor told me. For sure."

"Well, if that is true, that is rare, and we would be very grateful for a sample like that."

Suddenly, something that had caused us only pain seemed like it might have a higher purpose. I resolved to make this donation happen.

Having first spent several weeks getting used to the surprising news that we were having twins, we spent the next several weeks trying to accept the strange reality that we were going to have two babies but only one surviving child.

At thirteen weeks, we learned that the twins were boys. Ross reminded me of our deal from the first night we met:

I would choose names for our sons. I resolved that their first names would be simply ones I liked, and that their middle names would come from my brothers: Thomas Ethan for Baby A, and Callum Mark for Baby B. (It wasn't until Callum was three months old that we realized his name sounded like an appetizer at an Italian restaurant; we dressed him as calamari for his first Halloween.)

At fourteen weeks, I was referred to a new doctor, Alfred Khoury. Dr. Khoury was the medical director and president of the Inova Fairfax Hospital Medical Executive Committee. My mother worked at the Inova health-care system, and asked him personally to take care of me. "I will treat her like my own daughter," he told my mom in an email.

Dr. Khoury is a white-haired, fatherly man with a straight-talking but kind and patient manner. He was not only the president of the high-risk maternal-fetal practice, but he was also the president of the Medical Executive Committee of Inova Fairfax Hospital. He is not a man who shies away from responsibilities, and I felt that I could trust him.

Dr. Khoury explained that a selective termination was not impossible, though we had been told it was. He knew of a place in Baltimore that specialized in complex twin pregnancies, and suggested that we meet with them to learn about our options.

And so at sixteen weeks we found ourselves talking to two specialists at the University of Maryland's Center for Maternal and Fetal Care in Baltimore: Dr. Christopher R. Harman, director of the Center for Advanced Fetal Care; and Dr. Ahmet Baschat, director of Maternal-Fetal Medicine, who would later become director of the Center for Fetal Therapy at Johns Hopkins.

I knew from reading about the Center for Advanced Fetal Care that they'd had a lot of experience with complicated, and in some cases experimental, procedures; they'd been doing it for over thirty years. It seemed amazing to me what doctors were able to do to tiny fetuses in the womb. At the center they were able to perform surgeries in utero, including things like laser surgery, blood transfusions, fetal heart failure treatment—they could even insert a little balloon into a tiny baby's trachea to aid in lung growth. (The balloon is inserted at around twenty-six to twenty-nine weeks and then taken out at thirty-two weeks so that, once born, the baby can scream and breathe all on its own.)

On a video about the center on its website, Dr. Harman said something that stuck with me: "We're constantly reminded that pregnancy can turn out well, regardless of risk factors." Well, here we were, with risk factors. We were desperate to hear what Drs. Harman and Baschat would say, especially if it included something about things "turning out well."

First we met with Dr. Harman. He explained that Baby A, now known as Thomas, could pose a risk to Baby B, Callum. We learned that in some cases, mono-di twins share some blood vessels—a condition called twin-to-twin transfusion syndrome. That meant that my blood flowed to one of the babies, and then the blood flowed from that baby to the second baby rather than directly from me. If our twins had TTTS, and Thomas died in utero, which was a distinct possibility, it could kill Callum or leave him with cerebral palsy due to a loss of blood pressure. Not only was a selective termination possible; it was something that would protect Callum's brain function and ensure his survival. But as ever, it was our choice.

Dr. Harman explained how it would work. Cord occlusion, as it's called, would involve a metal tweezer-like instrument being inserted through my belly, where it would then grasp and cauterize the umbilical cord. This would cut off the blood supply to Thomas quickly and safely—safely for Callum, that is. Thomas would die in my uterus and stay there until Callum was ready to be born a few months later. Thomas's remains would collapse, shrink, and calcify, though they, too, would be delivered when Callum was born.

But there was a big problem: The doctors couldn't determine whether the twins had TTTS until twenty-two weeks, but the ideal gestational age at which to do cord occlusion is *before* twenty weeks. Past twenty weeks, the diameter of the umbilical cord is larger, and the instrument that is required to grasp the cord therefore has to be much larger. This makes the procedure way riskier: it can cause preterm labor and rupture of membranes, so it's not recommended.

Ross and I agonized for days about whether to let nature take its course or to pursue a medical intervention that could improve the odds of having at least one healthy baby. My head was filled with questions: What if we don't terminate? And what if Thomas dies in utero and Callum ends up with cerebral palsy and is never able to walk, or drive, or work? Could I look Callum in the eye and tell him, "I could have done something that would have prevented your disability. But morally, it made me uncomfortable, and that is why you will never be able to walk. Sorry." A selective termination seemed like the right thing to do—for Callum, at least—but these were incredibly difficult decisions to make.

Eventually, we made an appointment to have the procedure.

My parents were raised in large Catholic families, and I was wondering what my family might think about my having an abortion under these circumstances. When I brought it up with my mom, she suggested I talk to a priest: she thought that some priests would understand my situation and support our decision. And although I didn't feel that I needed the approval of a Catholic priest to do anything, I thought I would give it a try for my mom's sake. Through a friend, my mom connected me with a priest called Father Frank. In the phone call I explained the medical procedure and asked if he would perform a blessing.

"You don't know for sure if they have TTTS? You don't know for sure that there is a threat, correct?"

"No one knows. We won't know until twenty-two weeks, but we have to have the procedure before twenty weeks. What I'm telling you is all the information the doctors have available."

"If the twins are born next week, I can perform a baptism."

"You don't understand," I said, trying to remain as calm as possible, even though I could guess where this was going. "No one is being born next week. Thomas will die, and he will stay in there. His remains will come out in March with Callum."

Father Frank was silent for a bit. Then he said, "I would not be able to do a blessing, no. But when your other son is born, I could perform his baptism."

Thanks, but no thanks. Annoyed at myself for even giving this guy a chance, I thanked him for his time and said good-bye. I didn't need a priest to tell me my son is going to heaven. I thought, *Forget any religion that doesn't understand the medical situation.* Father Frank had demanded information that is not available in the real world. But more than that, this was not a hypothetical brainteaser—this was my real life. Lots of people were willing to help me—friends, doctors, acquaintances, and people I had just met on the Internet. Father Frank was not, and I didn't need to invite someone like that into my life if he was going to make my situation worse.

I told my mom that speaking to Father Frank had been a waste of my time, and worse—he had made me feel terrible. Undaunted, she asked me to try one more priest.

"Okay," I said, "but this is the last one. Really, I'm done."

Through another friend of a friend I met a priest called

Father John, and straightaway he surprised me. He listened intently to my story, and then he came up with a fully thought-out plan: because the procedure was being done with the intention of saving Callum's life, he would do the blessing. He quoted the Doctrine of Double Effect, attributed to Thomas Aquinas and colloquially also known as the Trolley Problem. Simply put, the doctrine argues that it's okay to do something that causes harm *as a side effect* if it ultimately causes something good to happen. (The Trolley Problem is an example of this "double effect": there's a runaway trolley, and you have the chance to divert it away from five people tied up on the line [a good thing], but to do so would kill one person tied up on the other line [side effect].) Father John said that since cauterizing the blood vessels was being done to protect Callum, the termination of Thomas's life would be a side effect. If a miracle happened and the doctor was able to cauterize the cord, therefore protecting Callum and Thomas survived, we would be happy—not sad. This act of cauterizing the blood supply was therefore morally defensible, and he would perform the blessing.

I had gone for a sonogram on my twins. Now I was wrestling with philosophy and Thomas Aquinas and five fictional people tied up on a trolley line.

The night before the appointment to terminate Thomas, the atmosphere at home was heavy. Ross was drinking a single malt and doing something I had never seen before: crying. We didn't want to end Thomas's life, even if it was to protect Callum.

I wrote this in my journal:

"I hope God is watching over the doctors tomorrow and protects me and Baby B, and makes it as painless as possible for Baby A. We named Baby A Thomas Ethan. I looked it up today, and Thomas means 'twin.'"

The next morning, we got up at 6 A.M., and Ross carried our overnight bags to the car in the dark. We had booked a room at the Marriott on Pratt Street, across the street from the hospital, so I could rest after the procedure and be monitored the next day.

Once we'd checked in to the hospital and were waiting to be admitted, I texted Father John to let him know everything was still a go. He texted back that he was visiting a family in another part of the hospital but would meet us at the Advanced Maternal and Fetal Care department as soon as possible.

"Sarah Gray," the nurse called.

We were led to an empty operating room, and I was given a gown. Ross sat on the chair next to the hospital bed as I changed and pulled myself onto the bed and lay down.

Dr. Baschat came in and placed the sonogram on my belly. He pressed harder, from more angles. He pressed and pressed, looking confused. Then he spoke:

"The baby has moved behind the placenta."

"What?"

He sat back on the stool. "The location of your placenta is now blocking where I need to do the surgery."

"So what does that mean?" It seemed like nothing was straightforward, not even this terrible procedure.

"Imagine the placenta is the size and shape of a paper plate. It needs to be here [he held out one hand] and now it's over here [he held out the other]. This is dangerous, because the placenta is highly vascularized, meaning it's filled with blood. This is good for the babies, but if I even nick it with my instrument, it will bleed."

"So . . . what are we supposed to do?" I asked.

He paused. "*Why* do you want to do this?" he asked, hesitantly.

"We don't!" Ross and I both laughed. "We thought it was the safest thing for Baby B."

"Well, that has changed. This is no longer safe for you. If you were my wife, I would not do this."

And with that, the decision was taken out of our hands. Ross grabbed my hand and held on hard. The doctor excused himself, I put my clothes back on, and we left the exam room. Father John hadn't arrived yet. I was dizzy with relief. I sat in the lobby and texted him to cancel.

Ross and I stepped inside the elevator to the parking garage. As the doors closed, we clutched each other.

I would carry both babies to term.

CHAPTER THREE

Better Than Nothing

O nce the decision was made to carry both babies to term, Ross and I set about our lives as best we could. We began slowly acquiring hand-me-down baby items, and changing our guest room into a nursery. We were afraid to prepare too much, thinking that we might further jinx the pregnancy. Each time we referred to an event that might happen postbirth, we used a disclaimer: "If this works out, and if we really do have a baby, we should [*fill in the blank*]."

I even felt guilty opening a book of baby names. Although we had names chosen, Ross and I referred to the twins as Baby A and Baby B up until they were born, just out of superstition. We learned to assume nothing.

In addition to *sort of* preparing to have a baby join our home, emotionally I had to brace myself for the heartbreak of losing a child at the same time. I was going to need all the support I could get during this pregnancy. My job offered an employee-assistance program that included free counseling, so I started seeing a grief counselor, Sheila, when I was three months pregnant.

I saw Sheila once a week throughout the pregnancy (and for

a short time after). Sheila provided a safe place to put the feelings I'd accumulated during the previous seven days. She explained that one of the ways to understand grief was to think of it in stages—denial, anger, bargaining, depression, acceptance—and how it was normal to flip back and forth between emotions.

I told her about the moments when I felt guilty for looking forward to Callum's birth because it meant that Thomas's death would be near, and other moments when I felt guilty for dreading Thomas's death because it came alongside Callum's birth.

Also, I felt betrayed. I had thought that if I was a decent person and followed the rules, my life would go as expected. I graduated from high school and college, I had a good job, I paid my bills on time, I stayed out of trouble. What did I ever do to deserve this? Sheila recommended I read *When Bad Things Happen to Good People,* by Harold Kushner.

Even as I spilled my guts to Sheila every week, I didn't cry that much. It felt empowering to tell her about my feelings, and I remember laughing and feeling happy during our sessions. But there were also moments when I felt sorry for myself. One day I was driving home from a conference and I was stopped at a red light. There, on the corner, was a man standing with what appeared to be three-year-old twins, one tiny hand in each of his. *That's what I'm supposed to have,* I thought. I lost it.

But there was very little relief in crying. It felt unhealthy, like when you're lonely and you go back to an old boyfriend because he's available, not because he's good for you. It didn't help me grow; it just kept me treading water in the same stagnant pool of negative emotions and self-pity. I started to realize that none of us is really "supposed to have" anything. When we are born, we are not presented with a warranty guaranteeing that everything will be great, or with a list of things we are entitled to. Life is more random than that.

At my job, I worked with people with severe disabilities, whether due to a genetic condition, disease, or injuries from accidents or combat. Some of these people would never be able to live alone, drive a car, get married, or have a baby. Bad things happen to good people for no reason; I saw it every day.

Thanks to Sheila, I also started to see that I could feel both happy about Callum and sad about Thomas. I didn't have to pick one. Just knowing I had an appointment with her each week reassured me in a way, like knowing that someone will collect the garbage that's been piling up in front of your house every Monday morning.

Once I was showing, I no longer had a choice about keeping the pregnancy to myself. And so I joined the ranks of so many pregnant women before me, facing the enthusiastic friends and strangers wanting to share the joy of my having a baby and exclaiming things like, "You must be so excited!" Or asking, "Do you know what you're having?" Telling someone I was having one healthy boy and one boy who would die almost immediately would be awkward, even if it was the correct answer. Usually I just smiled and explained that we were having "a boy."

I did share the truth sometimes, when it seemed appropriate. When I went on bed rest, I had to tell HR, and there were a few acquaintances who pressed me on why I was seeing doctors in inconvenient locations. I received an array of awkward responses: "You should just be happy that there's one," or, conversely, "I'll say a prayer for you. Miracles happen."

Not this time; no, not this time.

The truth was, the looks on people's faces when I told them made the whole experience even scarier for me. It was bad enough for Ross and me to go through this, but we could prop each other up as we went through this journey together, reas-

suring ourselves that we'd be okay. And then we'd turn around
and there would be friends and family crying and wringing
their hands, and we'd have to calm *them* down, all the while
convincing ourselves that our situation wasn't as dire as their
reactions made it seem.

At other times, it really did feel that dire, like I was about to
be eaten by a monster and everyone around me was shouting,
"Look out! It's a monster! Run away!"

But I couldn't run away. I had to accept it and find a way to
move on.

At the same time, I knew I had much to be grateful for. Yes,
I was jealous of people who had a normal, happy pregnancy.
But I also knew people who had it a hell of a lot worse than
me. I had a loving family and husband, a comfortable home,
supportive friends, a job I enjoyed, health insurance, clean water
to drink via efficient indoor plumbing, and I was still pregnant
with one healthy baby. That's more than some people ever have.
I still had a lot to be grateful for.

I loved feeling the babies kick; it was like having two
large guinea pigs wiggling around in the front pocket of a
hoodie. Thomas was at the bottom and Callum was on top,
so I could tell who was doing what. I had more sonograms—
approximately one every week for twelve weeks—than most
expectant women, who might have three or four during their
entire pregnancy, so I had the opportunity to witness what the
boys were up to regularly. We saw Callum suck his thumb. We
could see the babies kick each other in the face. One night I
felt a strange sensation that I hadn't experienced before, and
then I laughed when I figured out it was a hiccup. How neat
that the babies were big enough to do their own thing and
hiccup.

In an effort to keep a little positivity and humor going, I

set up an email account for Callum so that he could "correspond" with his dad. It was silly and filled with inside jokes and horrible puns, but it was also a way to remind us that there was something wonderful on the way amid all of the sadness.

Date: Tue, 17 Nov 2009
Subject: Hello from Callum Gray
From: Callum
To: Ross

Hi Dad,

Mom made me my own email account. Who knows if I will ever need it, but she wanted to reserve it anyway. You can contact me through this email address, or I can be reached in my mom's belly pretty much anytime. LOL!

Love,
your son Callum

Date: Wed, 18 Nov 2009
From: Callum
To: Ross

Hi,

Hope you are having a good day at work. Make a lot of money so I can go to a decent day care please. Also please learn how to fold and unfold a stroller. I could hear what happened at Babies R Us and it was appaulling.

Love, Cal

On Wed, Nov 18, 2009 at 11:22 AM, Ross Gray wrote:

Very good. By the way, your spelling is "appaulling"— must take after your mother.

From: Callum
To: Ross

Sorry about the spelling. I am negative zero years old and the size of a pepper. What do you expect? Give me a freaking break!

In time, I became accustomed to our new normal, and I decided that if Thomas's death was inevitable, at least it could be productive. If our suffering helped mitigate the future suffering of just one other parent, then that was better than nothing. We had already registered for the Duke study and hoped to be able to contribute, but nothing was guaranteed. Though the thought of the study gave us a little hope, there were logistics: if something happened during the delivery, or the cord blood wasn't collected properly, or there was a snafu during shipping, the blood wouldn't be usable.

Duke also requested that Ross and I submit our own blood samples. At one of my checkups, I refused to leave the doctor's office until the nurse drew my blood.

"I don't think I'm allowed to since it wasn't requested by my doctor, and your insurance probably won't cover it."

"It's fine, I'll pay for it myself."

The nurse still hesitated, but eventually I prevailed, although I think she drew my blood only so that I would go away.

Finally, with every task completed, my hopes got a little higher that the cord blood donation would be a success.

In December, Dr. Khoury told me that when it was time to deliver, I should have a C-section. Since Thomas's skull structure was compromised, his skull could be crushed by the pressure of being pushed through the birth canal. And even if he was delivered successfully—he would be first, since he was lower—there was always a chance that Callum could get stuck on the way out and I'd need a C-section anyway, so I agreed.

The procedure was scheduled for Monday, March 22, when the babies would be at thirty-six weeks' gestation—a few weeks early as a precaution, since it would be very cramped in the womb and that could stress the babies. (I understand that this is standard for multiple pregnancies.)

I was scheduled to go on bed rest shortly before the December holidays, when the twins would be at twenty-four weeks' gestation. Dr. Khoury recommended bed rest for all women carrying two or more babies, since humans weren't actually designed to have more than one. Mammals who carry litters, like cats, walk on four legs, which distributes the weight of the litter properly, he said. But since humans walk on two, there's too much pressure on the cervix.

The fact that I would be confined to the house for twelve weeks meant I had to get all of my prebirth errands done before Christmas. One of the most difficult was the day I went to a maternity store to buy a dress for the funeral. When I told the saleswoman I needed something black and formal, she suggested something with sparkle: "It's for a holiday party, right?" I couldn't bring myself to tell her the truth, and mumbled something about a work function. How would I explain that this was for a funeral of a baby who was not born or dead yet? I took a plain black dress into the fitting room. The woman looking back at me from the changing-room mirror exhaled and said, *Oh, God, this is hard.*

And just like that it was 2010. As the new year rolled around, I was home full-time, allowed to leave the house just once a week.

I loved it.

Thanks to my stockpile of sick leave, and the company's short-term-disability insurance plan, I received my full salary, so we didn't have to worry about money. Instead, I read books and I watched television. Friends said, "Aren't you bored?" No, not for a second. I so enjoyed being lazy that it was everything I could do to scramble to take a shower before 4 P.M., when Ross came home from work.

I was so big by then that I didn't want anyone to take pictures of me anymore. I struggled to find clothes that would fit, but since I was in pajamas most days, I bought only one or two outfits that fit my swollen middle on those rare occasions when I went out.

At the end of January, when I was seven months along, my mom asked if we were going to look into organ donation.

"When I raised the subject of donating Thomas's body to science with the doctor, he didn't think it was an option," I told her. I had been disappointed that the doctor said that, and I had thought that was that.

But Mom told me she had heard through the grapevine at work that a baby with anencephaly had died that week and that the baby's hepatic cells—liver cells—might be donated for transplant: "Apparently it's a new program. Do you want to look into it?"

"Sure," I said. "Let's give it a try."

My mom told me to call Becky Hill, the clinical-recovery

coordinator of the Washington Regional Transplant Community. WRTC is the federally funded organ-procurement organization—OPO for short—for the metro DC area. Founded in 1986, WRTC works with more than forty health-care institutions in DC, northern Virginia, and suburban Maryland. There are fifty-eight OPOs around the country, all federally funded and not for profit, from LiveOnNY, which services more than ninety hospitals in New York City and the surrounding counties, to Legacy of Life Hawai'i. Wherever you live, there's an OPO in your area. Physicians are asked to alert the local OPO when a patient has met clinical triggers that indicate a death is imminent (so the OPO can present the option of donation to the next of kin), but this does not always happen.

When I reached Becky Hill, I was struck right away by how sensitive and compassionate she was. She had obviously been through this process with families before, and it was a relief to talk to someone so experienced. She explained that Thomas's predicted size at birth would likely rule him out for donating to transplant, although there would be no way to know for sure until after he died. I told her about the liver-cell donation my mom had heard about, and she kindly said she'd look into it.

I imagined that when you died, all of your organs would be happily accepted, and I was surprised to learn that this is not the case. There are very specific criteria to donate organs. To donate for transplant, the donor needs to be free of communicable disease, and also must die in such a way that the donor's organs do not fail before they can be recovered—which usually means that the patient dies while connected to a ventilator. And the process that OPOs have to go through to make a donation happen is complex. After it is determined that a donation may be possible, the OPO presents the option of donation to the next of kin for authorization. (Most families don't make the first move, like I did, but then most families probably don't have months to plan for an expected death.) Then they evaluate the medical suitability of the donor for organ transplant, which has one set of rules, or for tissue transplant, which has another set, or for research, which has—you guessed it—different guidelines again. Then the OPO reaches out to the United Network for Organ Sharing (UNOS), the nonprofit organization that maintains a list of transplant recipients all over the United States, or to research organizations like the National Disease Research Interchange (NDRI) or the International Institute for the Advancement of Medicine (IIAM), or even directly to local academic institutions. Then that organization coordinates the recovery with one or more surgical teams for different organs and tissues, and finally transports the donation to its destination—and all of it has to be done fast, within just a few hours of death. The OPO often provides grief support services as well, including quilt programs and annual donor recognition ceremonies. (This is a part of the program I would come to know very well.)

In February, I was assigned a nurse, Kelly Gallo, from the Perinatal Concerns Program at Inova Fairfax Hospital Women's Center, where I would give birth to the babies. This is the same hospital where my brothers were born and the hospital system where my mom worked in the risk-management department. Inova Fairfax is considered one of the top hospitals in the Washington, DC, metro area, especially for gynecology and neonatology. They deliver around eleven hundred babies every year, and they have a level-four neonatal intensive-care unit—the level that can handle the most complex treatments and critically ill newborns.

Kelly Gallo's role was to help patients with complicated pregnancies and deliveries. She asked Ross and me to fill out a birth plan that would include instructions for Thomas's birth, with stipulations such as no ventilation, no vaccinations, and no antibiotic gel for his eyes.

I told Kelly that, if possible, I'd like someone to do a blessing over Thomas when he was born. Since Ross and I didn't belong to a church, Kelly introduced us in November to Philip Brooks, the staff chaplain for the hospital. Immediately we found him to be a calming presence: he spoke quietly and seemed truly at peace. He said he'd be happy to do the blessing.

I also told Kelly that we were interested in organ, eye, and tissue donation. She had never had a case of an anencephalic newborn who donated before, so, like Becky before her, she said she would look into it. I had already begun to realize that this emphasis on donation was helping me focus my thoughts on something positive. A terrible thing was about to happen, but I was building meaning around it. This helped.

Kelly talked to a neonatologist at the hospital, who told her that for donation the baby would have to be at least at thirty-six weeks' gestation, and four pounds in weight, and even then only tissue and bone would be suitable for transplant. Another doctor told her that the baby would need to be seven pounds but could donate retinas and liver cells. I suggested to Kelly that she reach out to Becky at WRTC, who told her what she told me: there was no way to know for sure until the babies were born. In the meantime, I could complete consent forms, get a blood test, and complete a medical and social history interview in advance of the birth—all in order to expedite the process. Kelly added to our official birth plan the request to call WRTC at the time of Thomas's death.

I was surprised by some of the things they asked about for the history questionnaire. Debra Goldstein, a family-service specialist with WRTC, met with Ross and me after one of my appointments at the hospital to fill it out with us. Before she began, she looked up from her clipboard and said, "These questions are personal in nature. They are the same kinds of questions you would answer if you were giving blood. Do you want to answer these in private, or do you want Ross to be here as well?" I said it was fine for Ross to be there, though I didn't quite realize the scope of what I'd be asked.

It started out easily enough, with questions about my job: Do you work near pollution or pesticide? Nope. General health: Do you smoke? Nope. Do you use intravenous drugs? Nu-ugh. And international travel: Have you ever traveled outside the USA? When?

Then the questions got kind of uncomfortable. Is Ross the father of this baby? Yup. How many sexual partners have you had? Have you ever had sexual contact with someone who was born in Africa? Hmm? The questions seemed just plain weird and beside the point, even though I understand now that they somehow related to the transmission of infectious disease.

Back then I was in a Zima-soaked college haze, I later joked with Ross. How was I supposed to know where all those people were born? This was pre-9/11; I was not checking passports.

Given everything, I supposed a few intrusive questions were hardly the worst thing we were going to face.

It was nearly time for Callum's arrival, and for Thomas's arrival and departure.

Ross called a funeral home to make advance arrangements.

"I'm so sorry, Mr. Gray. When was the death?" the funeral director asked.

"We don't know," Ross said. "He's not even born yet."

By March 10, 2010, we had to tell the hospital where to transport Thomas's body if he died there, as we expected he would. We found a children's cemetery in the DC suburbs, picked out a tiny coffin, and went over the list of mandatory expenses—cold storage, hairdressing, makeup; and the optional ones—a viewing ceremony, a limo ride for the coffin to the gravesite, a tombstone. A burial.

We tentatively scheduled Thomas's funeral service for March 29, six days after his predicted combination-birth-and-death day.

Twelve days to go.

CHAPTER FOUR

Hello, Good-Bye
March 2010

A few weeks before our scheduled delivery date, Ross received a letter from the U.S. Citizenship and Immigration Services (USCIS) informing him that his citizenship ceremony had finally been scheduled for Monday, March 22—the same day as the scheduled C-section.

We had waited more than five years for this appointment, longer even than we had been trying to have a baby. Obtaining Ross's citizenship had been a complicated and frustrating process, even though we were married. What would we do?

It had been a huge relief to finally receive the notice to appear at the naturalization ceremony, where he would take the oath of allegiance, even if the timing was supremely unlucky.

I called Dr. Khoury and told him about the conflict.

"We'll have to reschedule your delivery," Dr. Khoury said without hesitation. "Immigration will never reschedule. We'll do it on the twenty-third." I imagined he'd had some personal experience with USCIS, so quick had been his reaction to our news. Regardless, I was grateful for his flexibility, especially given how trying the whole immigration thing had been.

I had heard that immigration to America had been difficult enough before the events of 9/11, and after that it became even more so. I thought of the poem on the Statue of Liberty:

> Give me your tired, your poor,
> Your huddled masses yearning to breathe free,
> The wretched refuse of your teeming shore.
> Send these, the homeless, tempest-tost to me,
> I lift my lamp beside the golden door!

What an outdated relic those sentiments proved to be, at least for us.

Ross wasn't tired or poor when he arrived in the United States, but he would be by the time the USCIS was done with him. It took five years and about four thousand dollars in fees and a lawyer's help. Ross had to spend our first six months of marriage unemployed; he was not allowed to leave the country, but he was not allowed to work, either, even though he had a job waiting for him. Ross had a bachelor's degree in civil engineering and had been employed at an engineering firm in Glasgow. His company, Halcrow, coincidentally had a U.S. office near Washington, DC, so when he asked about the chances of moving to the DC office, he was delighted to find out that he would have a job waiting for him if he could work out his own visa. In fact, Halcrow merely wanted to know when he could start.

No such luck. I was embarrassed by how unwelcoming my country was to my beloved. Engaging with the USCIS was like dealing with the government of a third-world country. They were understaffed, and it showed.

The visa he eventually acquired was the K-1 visa, known as

the "fiancé visa." While he still lived in Scotland, he took a day off work and travel four hundred miles to the U.S. embassy in London to complete the required medical tests, including an HIV test, and a chest X-ray to prove he didn't have tuberculosis. It seemed bizarre and inhumane to not let someone move just because he has a disease, and well-known, treatable ones at that. We submitted photos of ourselves together and included receipts for all the phone cards we used to call each other. We were both required to write a letter explaining why we wanted to get married.

Once he moved to the United States and we were married, we had to provide further proof that we were a couple, including the details of our joint bank account, our shared finances, bills we paid together—you name it. We completed hundreds of pages of confusing forms, and then there were those thousands of dollars in government and lawyer fees. Ross completed a civics test with questions about American history and the American political system.

While all this was going on, we attended a wedding in Toronto. On the drive back, we were held at the border. Ross's visa had expired, and, the USCIS explained, there was a backlog in paperwork; so instead of issuing him a new visa, they provided a letter that would serve as his visa until the actual document arrived. The immigration agents in Buffalo, New York, didn't seem to be buying it, and asked us to step out of the car. We were forced to cool our heels for an hour while they figured out whether the letter was legit. I felt uncomfortable being treated as a second-class citizen, and it was unnerving to contemplate that my husband might not be allowed back into the United States. That ordeal had been a sharp reminder of what a jam I could end up in by cosigning a mortgage and having a family with someone who could be deported.

I wasn't able to attend Ross's ceremony because I was on bedrest, but my dad and my brothers, Mark and Ethan, did, and they all filled me in afterward.

About one hundred soon-to-be Americans and their family members met at the U.S. District Court for the District of Columbia. Most were dressed up, and it was a festive atmosphere, with balloons and American flags.

The future citizens stood, repeated after the judge, and became Americans. Afterward there were cookies, fruit, and soda, and the judge mingled with and congratulated the new citizens.

Ross had become an American on a Monday, and now, on the following day, he was about to become a father. He'd had quite a start to his week.

That Tuesday morning—March 23, 2010—I was surprised to find myself both happy and at peace. I was ready to stop being pregnant and be a mom. *Let's get this show on the road,* I thought. Ross seemed excited, too. When it came to facing Thomas's death, we were as ready as we were ever going to be.

After all the phone conversations with Becky Hill from WRTC to discuss donation possibilities and logistics, I finally met her in person when she came to see me that morning in the prep room. She looked to be in her late twenties or early thirties, and she had long, blond hair. She was holding a beige knitted blanket in her hands.

"It's nice to meet you!" she said with a friendly smile. "Our volunteers knit these comfort shawls, and we wanted to give this one to you."

"Thanks so much," I said. "I'm going to use this right now because it's kinda cold in here." Already in a thin hospital gown, I covered my bare legs with the soft, warm fabric.

Although I didn't realize it at the time, Becky and the

WRTC team had done some prep work that was unusual. Normally, WRTC arranges donations for adults and children. A baby who had not even been born yet was a new one for them. This presented some unique challenges. For starters, they were used to gathering data about a donor in the controlled environment of a hospital; trying to gather that information while the donor was still in utero was uncharted territory.

As she explained it to me, there are three general categories of donation: The first is for organ donation for transplant such as heart, lungs, liver, kidney and pancreas. Organ donation for transplant has the most stringent criteria and it changes as medical advances come along. Since organs need oxygen to function and people stop breathing after they die, typically the donor needs to have help from some kind of machine that can circulate oxygen through their body at the time of death. Organs are typically removed and on their way to be transplanted within an hour of the cessation of oxygen to the body.

The second category is for tissue donation for transplant (corneas, skin, bone, heart valves, tendons, ligaments, nerve tissue, blood vessels, etc.). Tissues do not need to be transplanted as quickly as organs. In fact, some tissues, such as heart valves, can be frozen for years.

Third is donation for research or therapy. If the organ, eye, or tissue is determined to be unsuitable for transplant (due to a lack of oxygen, positive test for a disease, having an unusual anatomical structure, or a variety of other reasons), it could be donated for medical or scientific research or a variety of therapies.

As we waited in the prep room, Becky told me that the organization that WRTC had in mind for Thomas's liver donation was Cytonet, a biomedical company in Durham, North Carolina. Cytonet had developed a protocol for transplanting liver cells into children with malfunctioning livers who are too small to receive a full organ transplant. The liver cells are injected as a bridge therapy to help the malfunctioning liver do its job until the children are big enough to go on the organ transplant list. Without this novel therapy, most of these children would die. The Cytonet option was the first opportunity WRTC had heard about for anencephalic infants, but, this, too, presented a new challenge. The recovery method was an unexplored area that fell between donation for transplant and donation for therapy: the liver had to be recovered within a certain time frame to remain viable, but less quickly than it would have to be for an organ transplant.

Cytonet required that donated livers be free from communicable disease, so WRTC needed a sample of my blood on the day of the birth to make sure I didn't have a disease like HIV or hepatitis that I might pass on to Thomas, which would rule out a donation to Cytonet. (Though diseased tissue is normally not suitable for transplant, it is extremely valuable for disease-specific research. In addition, after the Hope Act of 2015, a donor who is HIV-positive can donate organs for transplant to recipients who are already HIV-positive.)

On a good day, nurses can't find my veins. Because per C-section surgery rules I had not eaten or had anything to drink since midnight, I was dehydrated, and this made my veins collapse. The nurse was really struggling to insert a needle into the top of my hand, and was apologizing the whole time. She was trying to be gentle, but after numerous failed attempts my hand swelled up like a bear paw, and she left to find a colleague to help.

Ross was getting woozy.

"You don't have to do this," Becky said to me. "It's up to you."

"Let's forget it," Ross said. "It's not going to happen."

I looked at Becky. "But if I don't do it, we can't donate, right?"

She looked at the floor. "You don't have to donate."

"I want to donate. After all the work we have done? We'll get some blood."

The nurse came back with a doctor, the vein-finding ringer. Eventually, success! A vein.

"I'm sorry it took so long," Becky said, gathering up the tubes that now held my blood. "I'm going to bring this to the office now. I'll talk to you soon. Good luck!"

"Thank you," I said.

"No, thank *you*," she said.

Next, I was led to the operating room while Ross stayed behind. I was carrying a bag filled with test tubes that Duke had sent. "These are for collecting the cord blood. Where should I put them?" I asked.

A nurse put the bag on a table near the back wall.

"There are instructions in here, too."

"They know how to do it," she said kindly.

Even though this was now so important to me, I was still concerned that I was imposing. I understand that medical professionals care about one thing—the health and survival of their patient—and in this case, their job was to perform a complex surgery in a way that was safe for the twins and me. Asking them to collect cord blood for some study hundreds of miles away felt like asking a DC Metrobus driver to pull over at Starbucks and wait for me while I picked up my breakfast.

I'd never had surgery, so I didn't know what to expect. I'd pictured a small room with a window, like a normal hospital room, with a few hints of baby stuff like a stuffed animal here and there. Instead, the windowless room was at least three times the size of a normal hospital room. There were metal tables lining the walls, another room with two-way mirrors in the corner, and large medical equipment hanging from the ceiling. I had imagined that the bed would be the largest thing in the room, but in fact it was dwarfed by all the high-tech gizmos. The bed itself looked like nothing so much as a crucifix with a board on which to rest each outstretched arm. The whole thing was clean and sterile, with not a stuffed animal in sight; in fact, it had all the warmth and charm of mission control for a space flight. But if that's what they needed for a safe delivery, I could do without the stuffed animals. Looking around, I quickly realized that this surgery was no joke.

There were already a bunch of people quietly bustling about. One of them, a young woman in a white jacket, said, "I am a resident here, and I would like to observe the birth. Is this okay with you?"

"Sure, that's fine. Did they tell you about the twins?"

"Yes," she said.

I was glad to have one more medical professional learn something and witness what I imagined was an unusual case. There was no avoiding this bizarre situation, but maybe someone could learn from it. This young student at the beginning of her career added an element of hope for the future.

There must have been fifteen people I had never met already there, all dressed in scrubs, quietly going about their preparations. One of them, a man with an Eastern European accent, told me to bend over the operating table "like a rainbow" so he could administer an epidural. He told me to stay completely still while he inserted the long needle into my back. If I moved, I could paralyze myself. When I felt the sting of the needle pierce my skin, I let out a high-pitched "Ahhhhh!"

He told me I should try out for *American Idol*.

I had been afraid, and I was grateful for this silly comment that distracted me and put me at ease.

My legs started to feel tingly and warm.

"Hurry up! Get on the table!"

"Right now? Is this where I'm having the babies?" There was no reason I should know how these things go, of course, but nevertheless the surprises kept coming.

Dr. Khoury was stuck in traffic, someone said, so in the meantime they put a privacy sheet up so I couldn't see what was happening at the business end of the table. I felt someone lift my robe and, though I was numb to pain, I could feel the vibration of the electric razor as they begin to shave me. Given all the people in the room, I did wonder if they could all see me naked. With Ross confined to the waiting area until just before the doctor made the incision, I felt alone and lost, like I was at a party where I didn't know anyone.

Finally, Ross came in wearing scrubs and a mask.

"Am I naked?" I asked him.

"No, I don't think so," he said, "but I can't really see." Ross came to stand next to my head on my side of the privacy sheet and started taking pictures of us with our masks on; he seemed happy. Kelly, the nurse, and the chaplain, Phil Brooks, also showed up.

"Let me know if you feel like you're going to throw up," the anesthesiologist said from somewhere behind my head.

"Are you going to start the medication now?"

"I already started."

As he fiddled with knobs and equipment to administer the anesthetic, it sounded like he was chopping vegetables on a butcher block.

Suddenly, I felt Dr. Khoury make a painless incision across my belly from left to right. I hadn't even seen him come in.

Then there was a tug: Thomas, born at 10:32 A.M. I couldn't see him until they put him on a gurney over my left shoulder. He was small, just over four pounds, and covered in blood, but he was squirming and kicking his legs.

"Why don't you go see your son," Kelly said to Ross. Ross walked over to the gurney and picked him up.

I heard the chaplain say a prayer.

Then I felt another tug: Callum, born at 10:33, weighing in at five pounds, ten ounces. Kelly placed Callum next to his older brother, Thomas, on the gurney.

I was a mother. This was my family.

I heard Ross taking pictures. Then, out of the corner of my eye, I could see that something was wrong with Callum. One nurse was smacking his feet while another held a tiny oxygen mask over his face. We were all waiting to hear him cry, but nothing was coming out.

He was supposed to be the healthy one.

Just then, Kelly brought Thomas over to me and whispered, "His heart rate is dropping quickly." I knew what that meant: he was alive, but not for long.

She held Thomas near my head and I saw his face for the first time. I was relieved that he was actually born alive and we were able to meet each other before he died.

Thomas Gray had light brown hair in a circle around his head, like a balding man. From the nose down, he looked like a normal healthy boy. He had a cute, tiny little chin. Like the doctor said, he was missing the top part of his skull, and I could see some exposed red tissue on top of his head. One of his eyes was swelling and the other was closed. He looked scared and confused. His body language seemed to say, "What is going on? What am I doing here?" I thought, *This poor little guy. He has no idea what is happening to him.*

This was my firstborn son; this, the first time I ever saw him. And he was dying.

"I love you," I said to him.

"Can I touch him?" I asked Kelly, and she nodded. I stroked

his tiny cheek with my finger. This would probably be my only memory with him alive, and I wanted to remember it forever.

"Can I kiss him?"

"Sure."

I kissed my son on the cheek. I felt tears on my face, and I was overwhelmed by nausea.

Kelly took Thomas away and brought Callum.

"Here's Baby B. I think he looks like his mommy."

"Hi, little guy," I said. He did look a little familiar. "Why isn't he crying?"

"We don't know. We're taking him to the NICU now."

"Should I stay here, or go to the NICU?" asked Ross, starting to panic.

"It's okay, Ross, go," Kelly said. "Thomas's breathing is improving."

"Are you saying Thomas is doing better than Callum?"

"I'll be honest. Yes, he is."

Ross told me later he thought, *That's it. They're both going to die.*

Ross put Thomas down on the gurney and followed after the team that was running down the hall alongside Callum's gurney to the neonatal intensive care unit.

"I think I'm going to throw up," I said to Kelly.

"They're pushing on your uterus right now—that's why you feel like that." She handed me a little pink plastic tub.

Chaplain Phil Brooks stayed behind with Thomas. He told me later that he lifted Thomas out of the bassinet and held him in his arms.

"We talked for thirty minutes or so. I welcomed him to the world. Believe it or not, I was actually very centered and felt guided by the Spirit at that time."

Concerned that Thomas's condition might get worse,

Kelly and Phil then took Thomas to the nursery, where volunteer photographers Jay and Clarice Gibson, from the nonprofit photography organization Now I Lay Me Down to Sleep (NILMDTS), were waiting. The mission of NILMDTS is to take free professional photographs of babies with fatal diagnoses immediately following birth as a remembrance for the parents. Thomas got his picture taken with my mom, dad, and brothers.

Meanwhile, back in the OR, I started to feel really sick— like I was drunk, but in a bad way; the room was spinning. I vomited.

"Looks like last night's dinner," the anesthesiologist said. He gave me an injection of something in my shoulder.

"Give her Pitocin!" Dr. Khoury said. Pitocin is a synthetic form of oxytocin, the hormone that bonds mothers to babies and also induces contractions. They gave it to me to make my uterus contract to stop the bleeding from the incision.

"I already did," said the anesthesiologist.

"Put another one in."

I heard someone say, "Get a bag of blood." Then two bags. Then three bags.

Someone above me barked, "Code hemorrhage!"

"Where is the blood?" Dr. Khoury kept saying. "Did you call for it?"

"Yes, I called. It's on its way. I'll call again."

"I need it now!"

"I'll go get it," she said and left.

I imagined that Thomas had already died at this point. I imagined that Callum had brain damage since he didn't seem to be breathing. Was I going to bleed to death right there on the table, too?

I was growing weaker by the minute. I felt bad for Ross that all three of us might die in one day, or maybe I was going to leave Ross to raise a brain-damaged child on his own. I wondered how he would afford the mortgage; then I remembered my life-insurance policy and felt a little better. But since I handled our finances, I realized that Ross probably didn't even know the password to pay the bills online. I should have written down the passwords; so many passwords. Deathbed regrets for the new millennium.

I wasn't upset about dying. I thought that whatever came next would be better than this world, which was starting to feel like a festival of miseries.

"The blood is here."

I could sense relief among the people standing around me. I started to feel stronger, like I was waking up. Like I was alive. I later learned that I received three units of packed red blood cells, two units of fresh frozen plasma, one unit of cryoprecipitate, and one unit of platelets. (Cryoprecipitate is a concentrated form of plasma that helps with coagulation; it was originally developed for hemophiliacs but it's now used often during surgeries when a patient is hemorrhaging. One unit of this comes from five donors.) In total, I received blood donations from ten generous strangers.

The anesthesiologist said most C-sections don't take this long, but I was close to having an emergency hysterectomy. My uterus didn't contract when it should have to stop the bleeding after surgery. One reason might have been the fact that I had been taking Procardia, an anticontraction medication, for six weeks to prevent early labor.

"She lost *a lot* of blood," I heard Dr. Khoury say. "Okay. I'm going to go talk to the family."

Then I was done. I heard someone count: "One . . . two . . . three!" And they lifted me off the bed and onto a stretcher.

"Wow, that was just like on *ER*," I said, still woozy with anesthesia. The nurses gave me the red grocery bag filled with test tubes.

"Were you able to get the cord blood?" I asked. I had been afraid that in the drama something had gone wrong, or the nurses had forgotten to take the blood, or done it wrong, or something. Festival of miseries don't forget.

"Yes, no problem," a nurse said.

Yes! I was numb, floppy, and completely helpless, but when I realized that blood had been drawn, I felt like a Stone. Cold. Champion. I was wheeled out of the operating room feeling immense relief now that I had possession of these possibly valuable test tubes that represented all the hours of research and interviews and blood tests Ross and I had gone through.

I was rolled into a small recovery area that was curtained off for privacy. Ross came in, holding a bundle.

"Who is that?" I still felt foggy, like in a dream.

"Thomas," he said.

"He's alive?" I was delighted that our little guy had rallied and we would have a little more time with him.

"Yeah." Ross handed one of our sons to me. "We've been getting to know each other a bit." Ross had been able to spend some one-on-one time holding Thomas up in the nursery before he brought him down to see me in Recovery.

Thomas's little pink face nuzzled into my hair. He made little baby sounds. He wrapped all five of his tiny fingers around one of mine. I was delighted when he successfully breast-fed right there in the recovery room.

The nurses had put a soft blue hat on Thomas, but it kept falling off. I wondered if the hat would hurt his wound and decided to just leave it off. His appearance didn't bother me. I wished he was healthy, but he wasn't. After gaining forty pounds, going through surgery, and losing all that blood, I wasn't looking my best, either. Who was I to judge?

My family and the NILMDTS photographers showed up and started taking pictures in the tiny, crowded room. My brother Mark is a professional photographer, so there was a lot of posing and clicking. One of the things I thought was, *Everyone can see my naked boob.* But I didn't know how much time I had left with Thomas, and I was still on drugs, so I didn't really care. My family all seemed so serious, like they were holding back tears. Callum was still in the NICU, which was off-limits for the photographer, so Jay wasn't able to take any photos of the two boys together.

After a little while a nurse asked everyone to leave, and Ross and I were transferred to a private hospital room. Mark joined us there and took the test tubes of cord blood for Duke. He labeled them "Baby A" and "Baby B," packed them up, and dropped the package in the FedEx bin in the lobby of the hospital.

At some point a nurse came in and took Thomas's handprints and footprints. I was glad she did it so quickly; I figured we didn't have much time left with him.

I wondered how Callum was doing. Ross called the NICU, and I heard him say, "Yes, I am Callum's . . . father," a shrug and smile on his face as he tried on this new title for the first time.

When he hung up the phone, Ross said, "They're running some tests. He's doing okay. We can go down there and visit later."

In the meantime we watched Thomas, waiting for signs that he might die at any moment. But he didn't act as if he was dying at all; he seemed like a normal baby. He clutched our fingers, he breast-fed, he drank formula from a bottle, he went to sleep in the crook of Ross's arm, he peed, he pooped.

My boy crawled up on his elbows and put his head in the curve of my neck.

Meanwhile, I struggled to learn how to use a mechanical breast pump, which is as uncomfortable as it sounds. Colostrum is the thick, high-fat, high-nutrient, high-antibody breast-milk equivalent of butter that comes out when a baby is first born. It's a good first meal for a baby and has long-lasting benefits. Thomas got some of this since he was breast-feeding, but I used the pump so we could give some to Callum as well.

That evening, Ross wheeled me down to the NICU with the containers of colostrum so we could feed and visit Callum. The first time I saw his face after the birth, Callum's cheeks still had the impression of the strap that held the mask from the CPAP, or continuous positive airway pressure, machine that was helping him breathe. He blinked his dark eyes and shifted his glance from side to side, as if he were suspicious. The nurses recommended I give him skin-to-skin contact, which means getting the baby as naked as possible and holding him against as much of my skin as possible. Skin-to-skin contact has been found to calm babies, help regulate their body temperature, and expose them to safe bacteria. It seemed a little weird to take off his clothes and my gown right there in the NICU, surrounded by other babies and parents, but I did my best. He was still connected to some tubes, so we didn't go far from the incubator. He seemed to like the skin-to-skin enough, but he didn't quite get the hang of breast-feeding.

The next morning, Thomas had a seizure: his arms went to his side; his entire body tensed and then convulsed. He seemed to be holding his breath. *Here it comes,* I thought. This is the moment we'd been fearing.

We buzzed the nurse, Brandy Celnicker. I was grateful to hear that she had cared for a baby with this condition before.

"It's okay. This is normal for a baby with anencephaly," Brandy said. "This is how you fix it." She tapped him on the collarbone, and he calmed down. Thomas looked confused and scared as he caught his breath. His body language seemed to say, "What's happening to me, Mom?" I was helpless as he suffered. I wanted him to live, but not if he was going to be in pain the whole time.

During the next few days, my room was bustling with visitors, both social and professional, including our parents, brothers and sisters, and various in-laws, cousins, and friends. We also met with a grief counselor, WRTC reps, a genetic counselor, Phil Brooks, and my doctors. It was a strangely busy time.

Thomas continued to have tonic-clonic, or grand mal, seizures, increasing in frequency with each day. His doctor said that these might be caused by overstimulation—like bright light, loud noises, commotion, getting a bath—or even by being too cold. Whenever the seizures happened, we would tap his shoulder the way Brandy had taught us and hold him until he came out of it. Then I would breast-feed him or give him some drops of sugar water to calm him down.

With each passing day, it became a possibility that we might actually take Thomas home. Having expected Thomas to die within minutes of his being born, we were amazed that, four days later, he was still with us. I started to think, *What if he lives for a month? Or three months? Is he going to be the one who beats the odds?*

Do we need to secure day care?

Looking back, I remember something that didn't concern me at the time but now realize was a sign of what was to come. Ross and I had been asked to write down every time Thomas breast-fed or drank from a bottle. Because I was recuperating from the C-section and couldn't really get out of bed, Ross took primary responsibility for feeding, changing, and looking after Thomas, so he also took on the job of recording secretary. If Thomas drank from a bottle, Ross would make a note of how many milliliters he drank. The largest feeding he ever recorded for Thomas was seventeen milliliters, which is about three and a half teaspoons. Normal newborn feedings are recorded in ounces, a unit of measurement that is thirty times the size of a milliliter.

On day four, a nurse came in to check Thomas's meal chart.

"Did you guys forget to write down some of his feedings?"

Ross looked up. "No, we got them all."

"He hasn't been eating very much," she said.

"We have been trying, but he doesn't want to eat," I said. "He spits it out."

"Okay, just checking," she said.

There was one thing that Thomas seemed to like eating, and that was the sugar water we gave him after a seizure. My brother Ethan and I took turns putting some on his mouth and then watching him smack his lips. He sucked his top lip to get every last taste. We started asking visitors, "Have you seen him eat sugar water yet? Watch this!"

We learned that Callum was fine, just suffering from what is informally known as "Wimpy White Boy Syndrome." Male Caucasian babies are thought to take somewhat longer to develop than babies of other races, so when they're born prematurely, they tend to be weaker.

On Friday, two notable things happened. The first was that Callum was released from the NICU. The second was that I had to make one of the strangest phone calls of my life—to the funeral home.

"We have a funeral tentatively planned for Monday, but something unexpected has happened. Thomas was born alive, and he's still going strong. So we are going to need to postpone. Is it okay if I call you later?"

There was a pause. Then, "Yes, of course."

I had to postpone a funeral because the guest of honor was still alive.

Before we could take Callum home, Ross had to take him to the "Car Seat Challenge" in the hospital. This is a test where they put a baby in the car seat in a simulated ride to make sure the baby will be okay riding in the vehicle, and Callum aced it.

The minimum weight for a baby to ride in a car seat is five pounds. Thomas had lost weight since birth, down to three pounds, four ounces, so he didn't meet the criteria. The hospital gave us a special contraption, called a car bed, that is made for just this occasion. It is essentially a white plastic box that gets strapped into the backseat.

We were also asked if we wanted hospice care. It seems naive now, but I didn't fully understand what the term *hospice care* meant. I thought it was just a visiting nurse. It wasn't until later that I understood that hospice care is recommended by a doctor only when the doctor thinks the patient has less than six months to live and the patient has decided to die at home as comfortably as possible.

That Friday night, the four of us slept in my room in the hospital—our first night as a complete family in one place.

But we didn't get much sleep. I was nervous at the prospect of leaving the hospital and the round-the-clock access to experienced medical professionals who were available literally at the push of a button. I was not sure what we would do with Thomas once we got him home. We hadn't planned for this.

But sure enough, on Saturday, March 27, 2010, we took the twins home from the hospital to our condo in Washington, DC. When we arrived, one of the hospice nurses was already at our door, buzzing to be let in.

The house quickly became chaotic with people visiting and

the door constantly buzzing with deliveries of flowers. I was grateful that our families were playing with Callum while Ross and I looked after Thomas.

Thomas grew increasingly listless. When I changed his diaper, he flopped like a ragdoll. The nurse prescribed morphine and antiseizure medicine for him. Because he was so small, we gave him the medicine in doses of a fraction of a milliliter.

When he hadn't eaten anything in an entire day, I panicked and mixed up some homemade sugar water, but he wasn't interested. I tried to give him breast milk with an eyedropper, but he didn't want that, either. I thought if he only ate more, he'd perk up. "C'mon, little guy," I kept saying.

I didn't understand that his loss of appetite was likely a sign that he had started dying. I wish I had figured that out instead of frantically trying to feed him. I thought there was something I could do to help him, but probably there was not.

It was just his time.

On Sunday night, he began wheezing at around 11 P.M. I called the hospice company, who connected me to the nurse on call, Cindi Carney. I felt guilty, because she said she lived in McLean, Virginia, which is about ten miles away from where we lived, and I didn't want to bother her so late at night.

"It's perfectly okay, Sarah. That's why I'm here," she said.

I told her about Thomas's labored breathing. "What should I do?"

"That sounds like end-of-life breathing."

I didn't know there was such a thing.

"I'm on my way," she said.

"I'm sorry it's so late . . ."

Cindi arrived with a laptop and a stethoscope. She listened to his breathing and his heartbeat and confirmed that the end was near.

Ross and I called our families, and people started arriving around midnight: my mom; my dad; Ethan; Mark, his wife, Jennifer, and their nine-month-old son, Matthew; Ross's mom, Pauline, and dad, Eddie; and Julia and Garry, Ross's sister and her husband, all in from Scotland—all came in the torrential rain. I called Becky Hill so she could alert the WRTC team that something might be happening soon.

Ross and I held Thomas on our bed, and Cindi monitored Thomas's heartbeat. Thomas would stop breathing for a minute, and then take a giant breath in. He was barely moving. Everybody was crammed into our bedroom.

Months earlier, Ross had said that he would not be able to hold a baby while it died. But over the months that followed, Ross had changed. He was quick to stand up for Thomas. It was Ross who wanted to make sure we gave him a name, a proper funeral, and a tombstone for Callum to visit. Ross memorized and recorded how many milliliters of milk Thomas drank. Ross enjoyed sleeping with Thomas in the crook of his arm, feeding him, and changing his diaper. Ross claimed that since Thomas didn't cry as much as Callum, Thomas must be the smarter and more sensible twin.

Thomas was Ross's pal.

At the moment of Thomas's death, we heard a cry from Callum's crib.

"He knows," said Pauline.

I looked at Cindi. "His heart stopped?"

"Yes." She pulled the stethoscope out of her ears and let it rest on her shoulders. She looked at her watch and wrote down the time. It was 1:45 A.M. on Monday, March 29, 2010.

Thomas was resting in Ross's arms when he took his last breath. He was our firstborn, and he made Ross become a father in more ways than one.

CHAPTER FIVE

Thomas's Ride
March 29, 2010

We passed Thomas's body around the circle surrounding our bed so each of us could hold him one last time and say good-bye.

"We are hoping to donate organs through WRTC," I told Cindi.

"Do you want me to call them?" she asked.

"Sure," I said. "Let me give you the phone number."

"I have it," she said.

After each of us had our moment with Thomas, the family left Ross and me to have a private moment with him in our room.

Eventually, we moved to the living room and placed Thomas in the car bed. Cindi told us that the WRTC van was lost and had accidentally gone to a different street with the same name. A few minutes later, though, our door buzzed and we opened it for a tall man in his late twenties.

It was the moment we would say good-bye, at least until the funeral a few days later. My family is not particularly

religious, but it seemed like a moment for a prayer, or something. I was emotionally drained, though. I felt like I was in
a trance. I couldn't make a decision or think of anything on
the spot.

"Everyone put a hand on him," my mom said. The van driver
waited patiently with Cindi at the dining table as the family
gathered around the car bed. My mom quietly said prayers she
had repeated for years as a child in parochial school—the Our
Father and the Hail Mary, followed by one I had never heard,
the Angel of God:

> *Angel of God,*
> *my guardian dear,*
> *to whom God's love commits me here,*
> *ever this day,*
> *be at my side*
> *to light and guard,*
> *to rule and guide.*

With tears in my eyes, I looked to the van driver. "He's
ready," I said.

"Would you like me to carry him, or would a family member prefer to do it?" he asked gently. It felt like a heavy burden
to have to make that decision.

I wasn't supposed to walk downstairs because of my
C-section, but I hoped someone else would step in. I looked at
Ross, and he shook his head no.

"You can take him," I said to the driver.

My brother Mark jumped in: "No, I'll do it."

I was so grateful.

Outside, it was pitch-dark and the rain was still coming
down in sheets. Ross and I stood side by side at the window

and watched as Mark carried Thomas's body down the hill from our building. He placed the car bed in the back of the van and stepped away. The man shut the doors and drove off.

We watched as Mark walked back up the hill in the rain.

Thomas had spent every minute he was alive with people who cared about him: his parents, his brother, our families, our doctors and nurses, chaplain Philip Brooks. This part of his life was now over. He was going out by himself now.

We knew that Thomas would be transported to Children's National Medical Center on Michigan Avenue NW, in DC, which is less than two miles from our home. In another unusual twist to the preparations, WRTC had made arrangements with Inova Fairfax to do the organ recovery, assuming that Thomas would die there. They subsequently had to scramble to make arrangements with Children's National as opposed to Inova Fairfax, which even at only eighteen miles away would have been too far to send him. (I learned later that this was an unusual and professionally brave request of them to make since Thomas had not been a patient at Children's.)

We didn't know specifically which organs or tissues might be recovered, although we knew there was a chance for the liver to go to Cytonet if it met the requirements. In my dream-world, I wanted WRTC to tell me that every single part of my son's body was incredibly valuable and interesting, and that the field of science was about to take a giant leap forward because of him. The happiness and amazement I felt when I touched his little fingers, his chin, and his toes . . . well, I wanted researchers to feel the same thing when they saw his pancreas, his kidneys, his heart valves, and his ocular cells.

Mark came back in, and we all hugged one another and cried. I was exhausted down to my bones. Everyone else seemed to be drained as well. They left Ross and me to get some sleep.

Around 10 A.M., after a brief, exhausted sleep, the phone rang. It was Becky Hill.

"I'm calling to tell you the recovery was a success."

"What does that mean? He got there in time?"

"Yes."

"What did they recover?" I asked.

"His eyes and his liver."

"That's it?"

I was disappointed they didn't need more, but two things were better than one or none.

"We tried to find more placements, but those were the only two we could arrange. His liver is going to Cytonet, and his eyes will go to research."

"Where will they go? Do you know?"

"Not right now, but you will be getting a letter. For now, he's on his way to the funeral home."

Again, the news about the donation made me feel like a champion. The planning, the blood draws, the paperwork, the interviews—it had all paid off. In the midst of the pain, I felt accomplishment, even a lightness. Later that day I got an email from Heidi Cope at Duke saying the blood had arrived in good condition. Yes! I had done what I had set out to do in making these donations happen, but it was still too early to know if it was worth it. It was encouraging, yes, but also somewhat anti-climactic because there was still no sense of what the donations might do in the long run.

That same day, I got a call from Cyndi Barnett, a woman in Missouri City, Texas, who was pregnant with fraternal twins, one with anencephaly. When I was in the hospital, Heidi Cope had asked if she could share my contact information with Cyndi so I could offer her some support or advice.

Now, less than twelve hours after my son had died, I was

being asked to help someone else. It was wonderful to be in such a position. Instead of pitying myself, I was being given the opportunity to be grateful for what I did have. My pregnancy was over; I had a healthy child. Although I was heartbroken that my other child had just died, I could finally stop worrying about and preparing for his death. Cyndi's nightmare was just beginning. I was grateful that someone could benefit from what I had just gone through, and so soon. Cyndi's call helped change my perspective that day, and it gave me a little room to think of my situation in a different light.

Thomas's funeral was held on Wednesday, March 31, 2010.

Ross and I had been dreading this day for seven months, but when I woke up that the morning, I felt okay. I knew what to expect. Compared with how I'd felt the past six months, the funeral didn't seem nearly as difficult as I'd anticipated. And yet, nothing could ameliorate the reality of what we were about to do.

I put on my new black dress, the one I had struggled to find back in December.

Ross and I brought Callum to Fairfax Memorial Funeral Home early so we could spend some private time with Thomas—our last moments together as a family of four. We arrived to find flower deliveries along with some thoughtful gifts. Cytonet had sent two fluffy teddy bears with blue ribbons. WRTC had sent a letter explaining that on that very day, March 31, Inova Fairfax Hospital was raising the "Donate Life" flag on their flagpole in honor of Thomas's donation, and they had enclosed a picture of it. WRTC had also sent "Donate Life" lapel pins and green rubber bracelets, and I fastened a pin to my dress and one to Callum's car seat.

Though we had picked the coffin out in advance, and we knew how small Thomas was, its diminutive size still took me by surprise.

In the viewing room, the open nineteen-inch casket took my breath away for a moment: it seemed so small in that big room. Thomas was dressed in the dinosaur fleece pajamas we had gotten for him and Callum, and he was wrapped in one of the matching blankets that my Aunt Jane and cousin Kate had made for the boys. The blankets were leopard print with blue trim, to match the fleece Snuggie that Ross had given me as a joke present for our anniversary.

Around his neck, Thomas was wearing two gold Mizpah necklaces, each a broken half of a coin with the inscription: "The Lord watch between me and thee while we are absent one from another." I had gotten two of them so Callum could keep the other half of one and Ross and I would keep the other half of the other.

He also had with him a small Bible from his grandparents Gray; a palm frond and coin from my dad; a DVD of photos from Uncle Mark (all technology is compatible in the afterlife); a letter from Grandma Gray; a letter from Uncle Garry and Aunt Julia telling him they had named a star after him; socks given to him by nurse Brandy; a letter and prayer from my mom; and a stuffed sheep from Aunt Julia (Callum had a matching one).

And his most favorite thing of all: a little container of the sugar water that he loved to drink.

Thomas Ethan Gray looked so beautiful and perfect that it was hard to believe the recovery had taken place. (I looked for signs of the surgery but saw none.) I wanted to take a picture of him, but Ross didn't want me to. After a few minutes, the rest of the family arrived and joined us to pay their respects.

The funeral director, Adam, arrived and gave us his condolences. I thanked him for making Thomas look so beautiful. He asked if we wanted the pajamas he was wearing when he arrived (yes) and the car bed (no).

Adam escorted us out and placed Thomas in the back of the sedan for the drive to the Garden of Angels, a section of the Fairfax Cemetery just for babies. Thomas's spot was to be next to a tree that babies' families had decorated with wind chimes.

Phil Brooks had agreed to lead the service. When I'd asked him, he'd said, "It would be an honor. I haven't been asked to do a service in six years."

But what do you say about a six-day-old infant? We barely knew him and he was gone. Ethan provided the following notes to Phil, which he used to prepare his remarks:

Loved sugar water. Everyone enjoyed watching him lick and smack his lips.

Everyone who met him, family, friends, and the nurses all thought he was very friendly and loved him right away.

Although he was very small, he was strong. When he was only days old he would grab your finger with such amazing strength to come out of a baby of that size. He also beat the odds. He was only expected to live a few hours. He lived for 6 days, which gave all of the family time to let him know how much we loved him and cherish him. He wasn't supposed to be able to swallow, drink from a bottle or hear, but he could. He could also hold his head up and he would crawl up his mom's chest to her neck to chew on her hair. He had a 10% chance of coming home but he beat those odds and made it home. It is as if no one told him that he had anencephaly. He was very alert, strong, began breast-feeding before his brother, and very willing to make it known that he wanted more sugar water.

Sarah and Ross both were able to sleep with him not only in the hospital but at home as well.

He is now an angel looking over and protecting his twin brother, Callum.

He loved both his parents, especially Ross. Except once he peed in Ross's armpit during a diaper change. Ross didn't realize it at first and just thought he was sweating.

In his short life, he was photographed by Uncle Mark relentlessly. There are over 1,500 photos of Thomas.

In his short life, he made a difference in the lives of others. He was able to help the Duke University Anencephaly study. Duke is researching anencephaly and Thomas and Callum (and Sarah and Ross) both donated blood to further the study. Also Thomas donated liver cells and his eyes to the Washington Regional Transplant Community. The liver cells will be used by other babies who need a liver transplant and are waiting for a donor. So Thomas will continue to live on in other people and in the hearts of the people who loved him so much.

He died at home surrounded by family: Ross, Sarah, grandparents Suzanne and Jim, Eddie and Pauline, Uncles Mark and Ethan, Aunt Jennifer and cousin Matthew, Uncle Garry and Aunt Julia.

Phil then read the famous bereavement poem attributed to Baltimore housewife Mary Elizabeth Frye, thought to be the only poem she ever wrote:

> *Do not stand at my grave and weep.*
> *I am not there; I do not sleep.*

I am a thousand winds that blow,
I am the diamond glints on snow,
I am the sun on ripened grain,
I am the gentle autumn rain.
When you awaken in the morning's hush
I am the swift uplifting rush
Of quiet birds in circled flight.
I am the soft stars that shine at night.
Do not stand at my grave and cry,
I am not there; I did not die.

Then it was time.

We watched as Thomas's casket was lowered into the ground, and we all tossed white roses and lilies on top. Ross and I were so proud that we could give our son such a beautiful send-off. It was exactly right.

After the funeral, we went to Mark's house in Alexandria for lunch. It was such a lovely day that we ate outside on the porch. Mark showed a five-minute photo and video montage he had made of Thomas. I was so grateful to him for taking all those pictures and spending all those hours making the video. I was especially happy that my stepmother, Cathy, was able to see it. She had been sick and so hadn't been able to meet Thomas in person; the video made her feel like she got to know him after all.

Later that day, Ross and I and Callum went back to our house to begin our life as a family. I took a nap with Callum on my chest, and Ross went for a run—something he often did to clear his head after a long day at work.

The worst two days were behind us.

In the days after the funeral, Ross and I tried to make the transition back to the normal life of new parents. It was such a blessing to have Callum, who was now a healthy little guy.

We sent out this bittersweet birth announcement:

Dear Friends,
 It is with great joy that we celebrate
 the birth of our son
 Callum Mark
 Born March 23, 2010 10:33am
 19 inches, 5 lbs, 10 oz.
 We are deeply saddened by the loss
 of his twin brother
 Thomas Ethan
 15 3/4 inches, 4 lbs, 1 oz.
 Born March 23, 2010 10:32am
 Died March 29, 2010 1:45am
 He had a fatal neural tube defect called anencephaly.
 For those who would like to donate in his honor,
thank you. Our family participated in this research to find
a cure: http://www.chg.duke.edu/other/giving.html
                                    Sarah and Ross Gray

When Callum was six weeks old, Ross and I spent a long
weekend in the Bahamas visiting with one of Ross's college
friends, Scott, who was working there on a civil-engineering
project, and Scott's girlfriend, Justina. After three months on
bed rest in the dead of winter and the "snowpocalypse"—as
the media called the seemingly endless string of blizzards that
hit the East Coast that year—it was wonderful to be in the sun.
While we were away, my mom and dad got to exercise their
grandparent muscles and took turns babysitting Callum.

 In June, I went back to work and Callum went to day care.
I still went to grief counseling once a week. Ross handled the
loss of Thomas in his own way—getting on with life and keep-

ing up with the needs of a new baby. Between his obligations to work and to our surviving son, if Ross had any down time, it was for sleep or to go on a run. For him, there simply wasn't time to dwell on the loss.

I came to realize that we should have no expectations about how long we will live. People say, "No parent should have to bury a child," but there is no *should* in life. Just because one person lives to ninety-five doesn't mean everyone else is guaranteed the same. There is no one in charge, making sure that we all get our fair share of days or years. Children have been dying before their parents for millions of years.

However, I liked to imagine that Thomas had gone to the "other side," and that he was happy there. I imagined that Thomas did not pine for us, that he didn't want us to make a big deal about his being gone. He wanted us to be happy, because he was. He had new friends on the other side, and we would see him later. That was good enough for me.

Until it wasn't.

Before long, I started to feel like a piece of the puzzle was missing.

ELI'S STORY

Jodie and Jesse McGinley thought they had their lives figured out. They had good jobs, a nice home, a wonderful marriage that began with love at first sight—everything just as it should be.

So when the McGinleys decided to start a family, there was no reason to think that this part of their lives wouldn't go smoothly as well. Then Jodie suffered a miscarriage. They were heartbroken but determined to keep trying, and eventually they sought the help of a fertility specialist. Jodie endured months of painful treatments before she finally became pregnant, only to miscarry again. Beginning to think adoption was their only choice, the McGinleys decided to give in vitro fertilization a try. It worked. On Christmas Eve 2008, an ultrasound revealed that Jodie was pregnant with twins.

The McGinleys were ecstatic, but given Jodie's pregnancy history, they were immediately referred to a high-risk-pregnancy specialist at the University of Arkansas for Medical Sciences (UAMS) in Little Rock.

For the next few months, the doctor kept a close eye on Jodie. Regular checkups and ultrasounds were joyful times, if not without a few scares. A complication during the first trimester resolved itself; another complication during the second terrified them, but they got past it. When it was time for the twenty-week ultrasound, at which they would be told the sex of the twins, Jodie and Jesse brought their parents with them to the appointment to share in the excitement.

As the tech moved the wand over Jodie's expanding belly, she said, "Baby A . . . it's a boy. And Baby B, too!"

"I always wanted a boy," Jodie said. "It was a great moment," she later recalled.

But then the tech left the exam room to fetch the doctor. They thought nothing of it. The McGinleys and their parents were still celebrating the news when the doctor came in and put his hand on Jodie's knee.

"We have to talk," he said.

That's when Jodie's world stopped.

Baby A had the most common neural tube defect: spina bifida, which affects approximately fifteen hundred babies each year in the United States. With this condition, the backbone doesn't form properly in utero, so the spinal cord is exposed and often becomes damaged. Unlike with anencephaly, babies with this condition are not doomed to certain death, but it does result in physical and intellectual disabilities that can be anywhere from mild to severe, depending on where the opening in the spinal column is: up high near the head, paralysis of the legs can result, requiring the patient to use a wheelchair; lower down, the patient might have more use of the legs and get around with braces, a walker, or even no extra assistance at all. Incontinence is often a problem, and a catheter may be required as the child grows up, or even surgery in severe cases.

If the spinal cord is exposed, the first step after birth is surgery to close the hole. Babies with this defect may also develop hydrocephalus, also known as water on the brain. Since infants' skull plates are still separate, the accumulated water causes the head to swell and expand to make room. In addition to the disfiguring effect, the condition can also result in permanent brain injury, so a surgeon may install a shunt to drain excess fluid. (Babies have an advantage over adults when it comes to treating hydrocephalus: in adults, the skull is rigid, so there is no ability to make room for excess fluid, which rapidly leads to a severe pressure buildup that can cause brain damage and even death unless surgeons perform a craniectomy—the removal of a portion of the skull—to relieve pressure. The removed portion of the skull is often implanted in the patient's abdominal wall for safekeeping until the swelling goes down and the skull section can be replaced.)

Jodie worked with special-needs children, so when the initial shock of the diagnosis wore off, she realized she knew what to expect. They left the doctor's office in tears, but full of plans for the two new lives that would be joining their family in a few months. "We knew this was a blessing, and we weren't going to let that get us down," Jodie recalled.

On August 3, 2009, Jodie, at thirty-six weeks along, delivered her boys, Elijah and Walker, at UAMS. Eli, the baby with spina bifida, was the larger twin, weighing in at six pounds, three ounces; Walker was five pounds, seven ounces.

Jodie was able to see her children and touch their hands before they were whisked away. As planned, Eli was placed on a ventilator and transported by ambulance to Arkansas Children's Hospital (ACH), about two miles away, for evaluation. Walker was sent to the NICU at UAMS for observation. Jodie went to recovery.

Over the next two days, Jesse traveled back and forth between hospitals to see Jodie and baby Walker in one, and baby Eli in the other. On the second day, Jodie and Walker went home, and Eli went into surgery as expected to close up the hole in his spine.

And then an MRI of Eli's skull revealed what would change their lives forever. Eli had hydrocephalus damage, a herniated brain stem, and a Chiari 3 malformation, which is fatal. Eli would never be able to breathe on his own.

Jodie and Jesse had been anticipating bringing home one healthy child and one with special needs. It began to register that they would not be bringing home two children, but one.

They might not need that second car seat.

"Would he be eligible for donation?" Jodie asked. She didn't know where the idea came from. No one in either her or Jesse's family had ever received or donated organs or tissue. "I feel like the Lord just put the words in my mouth," she recalled.

A nurse practitioner offered to call ARORA—the Arkansas Regional Organ Recovery Agency. Reps from ARORA began research to determine whether he would be a suitable candidate. After a few hours, the McGinleys got the call verifying that Eli could make a gift of his aortic and pulmonary valves.

Surrounded by their families and their pastor, the McGinleys were with baby Eli when he was taken off the ventilator. The doctors had said that Eli would die shortly thereafter, but he survived another thirty-one hours. The medical staff arranged for Eli to be transported back to UAMS so he could be reunited with his brother, Walker, in the NICU. As the two babies lay side by side in their incubator, the pink returned to Eli's cheeks and a slight smile crossed his lips.

Jodie got to hold her baby and tell him how much she loved him. In his final hours, as his oxygen level started to decrease, Jodie whispered in his ear, "Come back to me. Just come back to me," over and over. She was asking him for reassurance that their decision to donate was the right one. Eli McGinley passed away in his mother's arms on August 8; he was five days old.

On Walker's first birthday, Jodie contacted ARORA for an update. Eli's heart valves had been sent to CryoLife, a biomedical company and tissue bank in Kennesaw, Georgia. Founded in 1984 with just six employees in a lab near the Hartsfield Airport in Atlanta, CryoLife was, by the time the McGinleys donated, at the forefront of cryopreservation technology, specializing in the low-temperature preservation of heart valves for children born with congenital heart defects. It is now an enormous, multinational company with more than five hundred employees and conducts business in more than seventy-five countries around the world.

Somewhere in its sprawling headquarters, Eli's valves were still waiting for a recipient.

A few days later, Jodie was under the weather, which she attributed to being sad about the first anniversary of Eli's death. Nine months later, on April 8, 2011, she gave birth to a little girl, Ellie Reese. Jodie calls her daughter her "rainbow baby."

Four months after *that,* on Walker's second birthday, Jodie reached out to ARORA again and was told that Eli's aortic valve had traveled north to a hospital in Maine, but there was no additional information.

It wasn't until December 1, 2014, that the McGinleys finally received an email from CryoLife telling them that Eli's aortic valve had been transplanted into a little girl the previous January. "I knew there was another mother out there who would not have to feel what I had felt. Just to know a piece of Eli was out there living took a big burden off my heart," Jodie said.

Jodie was busy preparing for a trip to Pasadena, where a floral portrait, or "floragraph," of Eli would be included on the Donate Life America float in the 125th annual Rose Parade on New Year's Day. He was only the second Arkansan ever to be so honored.

As soon as she returned home from Pasadena, Jodie was at her computer to resume tracking down her son's journey. Although fully understanding the rules of confidentiality surrounding transplant, Jodie wanted to know where the surgery had taken place, and anything else she could find out.

Then she did something both clever and extraordinary: She Googled "television news anchors in the state of Maine." *News anchors know everything,* she reasoned. In doing so she came across Kim Block, a longtime veteran anchor for Portland's Channel 13 WGME six o'clock news. Block specialized in medical reporting, so Jodie fired off an email. "It was a shot in the dark," Jodie said.

The next morning, Jodie received the most astonishing reply. Not only could Block help her; Block was friends with Dr. Reed Quinn, the Chief of Cardiac Surgery at Maine Medical Center and an adult and pediatric cardiothoracic surgeon, whom she had met while on a trip with Doctors Without Borders. Block offered to reach out to him on Jodie's behalf. Shortly thereafter, Dr. Quinn confirmed that he had indeed done the surgery and would let the recipient family know that the McGinleys would like to be in touch with them, if they were willing.

Nick Cates and Kiara Gadbois-Cates, a couple from Standish, Maine, discovered at their twenty-week ultrasound that the little girl that Kiara was carrying had a hole in her heart. At thirty-two weeks, they learned that their daughter's aortic arch would have to be reconstructed. At birth, baby Cambrie was taken straight to the NICU. They weren't able to hold her until the morning of the surgery at Barbara Bush Children's Hospital at Maine Medical Center. After about five excruciating hours, Dr. Quinn came out of the operating room and told them, "Our girl's doing great." He said that as part of the reconstruction procedure, Cambrie had needed to have her aortic valve replaced. "At that point it didn't click that another baby had passed away," Kiara said.

"You know, a donor tissue—that means another baby died," Nick said in the car on the way home. "That's a piece of another baby."

Many months later, Kiara was on her way home from work when she received a call from Lori Hafner, Dr. Quinn's nurse of twenty-four years, in the surgeon's office. "I have a question for you," Lori said. "The donor family contacted Kim Block, and Kim Block reached out to us. They'd like to meet you."

Lori arranged the phone call between the two moms.

That first call "was hard," Jodie said. "I was really choked up even thinking about talking to her." She even texted Kiara beforehand to say, "I just want to find the right words to say before I call."

Fighting back her swelling sense of panic, Jodie went into her bedroom, sat on the bed with Jesse, and dialed. When Kiara answered, the first thing Jodie noticed was her Down East accent.

"We were so excited and had so much to tell her. We were so emotional. We didn't think this would ever happen for us," Jodie said.

For her part, Kiara couldn't stop thanking Jodie and Jesse: "You saved our little girl's life."

Two months later, in March, the McGinleys traveled with their two children to Maine to meet Cambrie. "I thought she was the most beautiful little girl I had ever seen in my life," Jodie said. "She had really big, dark eyes and a head full of dark hair. I thought, *Okay, Lord, you knew exactly what I needed to see.* She was picture-perfect." Jodie put her hand on Cambrie's chest to feel Eli "pumping away in her heart," as Kiara put it.

It was remarkable that a baby boy who died one thousand miles away four years earlier had given a little girl he'd never met her future. What was perhaps more remarkable was the way the surviving children seemed to understand their bond. Walker was an energetic little boy who happily roughhoused with his little sister. But when Walker and Cambrie were together, he was extremely gentle with her—not just that he seemed to understand that she remained a physically delicate little girl, but that there was something special about her. "He's so good with Cambrie. With his sister, it's a different story," Kiara said.

And Cambrie put her chubby arms around Walker, hugged him hard, and told him she loved him. She was too young to understand their connection, but it appeared she felt it at some level.

"How blessed are we as the donor family to be able to watch Cambrie grow up!" Jodie said. "I couldn't ask for anything more."

Eli's pulmonary valve was the kind of donation that can be safely stored in cryopreservation for up to five years. If a tissue is not requested by a physician in this time, Cryolife may provide these life-saving tissues for humanitarian use in the United States and abroad and forgo the standard reimbursement of recovery fees. The McGinleys learned that Eli's pulmonary valve was shipped to the Dominican Republic in November of 2015 as a part of this program, called CryoKids. This valve was remarkably small, which made it less likely to find an exact size match for a transplant. However, a surgeon in the Dominican Republic was able to use Eli's tissue as a patch on the heart of nine-year-old Luis Angel Mercado on April 15, 2016. A photo of Luis and his family was shared with the McGinleys.

Six-year-old Walker looked at the photo of Luis and said, "Wow, how many times is my brother going to save a life? He's a hero."

CHAPTER SIX

Transplant Envy

The Washington Regional Transplant Community—a federally funded organ-procurement organization, or OPO—has, like many OPOs around the country, a dedicated donor-family support program that can continue for two years after a loved one's gift has been made. WRTC sends regular mailings about grief and loss, and proffers invitations to bereavement seminars and support-group meetings. These meetings are not exclusive to donor families, however; it is part of WRTC's charter to include anyone in the community who would like to attend, donor family or not.

In October 2010, Ross and I were invited to WRTC's Donor Family Grief Retreat. The retreat was held in a large conference room at the WRTC offices, making the atmosphere almost like a business meeting, with fancy sandwiches, snacks, and a Keurig coffee machine.

At the beginning of the retreat, the group leader asked us—there were about twenty-five attendees—to introduce ourselves and talk about whom we were grieving.

It was an eye-opening roll call:

"My name is Linda. My daughter, Jennifer, died of a gunshot wound. Her organs saved the lives of six people. We received a few letters from the recipients."

"I'm Sondra. My daughter, Felicia, died last year. She was a single mom, and she leaves behind her son, Daniel, who has special needs. I am taking care of him now, and he really misses her a lot. We all do. We donated her heart valves. She saved one life that we know of so far."

"Hi, everyone. I'm Marian. My daughter, Jessica, died in a car accident. She was twelve years old. We donated both lungs, her liver, and both kidneys. She saved the lives of four people." Marian's mother paused to compose herself. Then she said, "We received two letters of thanks."

I froze. But the stories continued.

"My name is Dave. My baby, Hannah, died in childbirth. My wife couldn't handle it, and six months later she committed suicide and donated tissue. So I am grieving two people."

As the stories continued around the room, I was in awe. I had never in my thirty-six years met one person who was involved in a transplant, and now I had just heard from twenty-five on the same day. I was impressed that these everyday people had directly helped save so many lives. And they received letters of thanks? It gave me the chills.

But when it was my turn to talk, the story didn't seem to compare. Ross felt the same way; somehow, perhaps because we'd known our loved one was going to die for months before it happened, and he'd been so young, our loss seemed less significant than those of the people who had lost spouses and older children who left behind a legacy of years rather than days. Also, we were the only ones in the room who had donated to medical research rather than to a life-saving transplant. All these people had the knowledge that they helped save a life; our effort was still theoretical.

"I'm Sarah," I said, haltingly, "and this is my husband, Ross. Our son Thomas died of a birth defect—it's called anencephaly—when he was six days old. His eyes and liver were donated for research, so he didn't . . . save any lives. But maybe he helped a study. Or something."

As I finished speaking, I found myself experiencing the most peculiar sensation: transplant envy. These people knew—or had the option to know—where their loved ones' donations ended up. I realized that if we had donated to transplant, we, too, might actually learn about the results of Thomas's gifts. But since we donated to research, the results would be much more mysterious.

Unknown, even.

Once the introductions were over, the counselor gave us each several exercises to do. We were to write letters to our loved ones, and we were tasked with writing letters back to ourselves from our loved ones. I wrote to Thomas and told him that I loved him and hoped he was having fun in heaven, and that if I won the lottery I'd know he was looking out for me. (It really would be an especially notable miracle, given that I never buy lottery tickets.) And then, as Thomas, I wrote back to myself to give myself a break: I told me that I didn't deserve what had happened, and acknowledged that I was doing the best I could.

Then the counselor passed out squares of aluminum foil with the instruction to make something out of it. I folded mine into a hat. Ross crushed his into a ball.

"Now crumple it up then try to make it flat again," the counselor said.

After a minute in which the only sound in the room was a faint crinkling as we followed instructions, he said, "Who preferred the part where you created something?"

I raised my hand.

"And who preferred flattening it out?"

Ross raised his hand.

"Some people like to create something new, and others feel more comfortable when they know what the specific goal is."

While it was grief that brought us together, there was also laughter. It was liberating to talk about death among strangers and not feel awkward. One man—whose brother was accidentally shot and killed—said that he found himself infuriated by the things people complained about in their lives on the social media he followed: *"My train was late,"* people wrote, or *"My computer broke."* Or *"My barista messed up my coffee order."* Losing his brother had made him realize how little these things mattered.

After hearing all these stories of loss, I felt lucky that Thomas had been just a baby with a disease. We hadn't relied on him to pay the mortgage or to pick anyone up from school, and we didn't face the chaos of emotions that result when someone takes their own life.

Through this shared experience, I felt that these people "got" me and what I was going through. All the normal small talk didn't seem necessary. I felt a level of comfort among these strangers that I hadn't always felt with my friends and colleagues since Thomas's death. I instantly cared about them and felt that they also cared about me.

Dave—the man whose story of an infant death followed by a suicide broke my heart—approached me during a break.

"I just want to tell you how sorry I am that you lost a twin. That must be so hard when you see the other boy."

And that's how Dave—a stranger, and a man who'd lost his child *and* his wife—told me he felt sorry for me.

Later, as we prepared to leave, one of the donor parents took me to one side and said, "It's really great that you donated to research. Who knows how many people your son's donations will help?"

"Yeah, who knows?" I said.

And I thought, no really, I would never know. Unless I got a letter, as some of my peers had.

WRTC, like all OPOs, protects the privacy and anonymity of participants. But that's not the whole story. After a transplant takes place, the transplant recipient and the donor's family can, if either party wishes, write to each other in care of WRTC. WRTC will forward the letter to the addressee along with a note that tells the recipient that if he or she isn't ready or willing to read the letter, he or she should either put it aside or return it to WRTC.

"We rarely get them back," said Lisa Colaianni, WRTC donor-family advocate and employee of more than twenty years.

If both parties decide that they would like to meet, WRTC facilitates the get-together (once both sides have signed a waiver form in accordance with the Health Insurance Portability and Accountability Act of 1996, that is). And those meetings can lead to bonds that last a lifetime.

Some people—on either side—are not interested in corresponding or meeting for a variety of reasons. One reason I heard from a recipient is that they are afraid that the donor family will not think they are "good enough" to receive their loved one's organs.

But some of the meetings are simply magical.

One such donor family–recipient meeting took place at LiveOnNY, the OPO in New York City.

LiveOnNY's Donor Family Services Aftercare Department organized a meeting between the family of a young Dominican man who had died of a cerebral hemorrhage and his heart recipient.

The donor left behind young children and a common-law wife. At the time of the donation, the common-law wife was not in the "order of priority" to authorize donation, and the donor's mother provided consent for the donation. (The order of priority in New York State has since changed, and since 2009 domestic partners have a say in the donation decision.)

The heart recipient was Dr. Anthony DiMaria, an internist at a local hospital in New York. After his transplant, the middle-aged doctor wrote to the LiveOnNY aftercare program, saying he wanted to contact his donor's family because he felt it was necessary, if possible, to thank them in person for the "generous gift of life that they had given me."

On the day of the meeting, the donor's six brothers and their wives and partners, all their kids, and the donor's mother gathered in a conference room—each excited and nervous to meet the man who had received their loved one's heart.

When Dr. DiMaria walked into the conference room where the family was waiting, the donor's mother was already standing with her arms open, waiting to receive him. She gathered Anthony to her and said, "*Mi hijo vive.*"

My son lives within you.

Soon, the rest of the family converged into a huge group hug.

"She said she wanted to feel the heart beating," DiMaria said. "I had my stethoscope." The family took turns listening to his heartbeat.

Then, it was time for a photo. As the donor family crowded around Dr. DiMaria, one brother playfully asked him if he had started to like spicy food. Another brother, himself a kidney transplant recipient, said, "Now we are seven brothers again."

To this day, Dr. DiMaria keeps in frequent contact with one the brothers and sends flowers to the mother and her family on Mother's Day and Christmas.

"I tell people I am Italian-American with a Dominican heart," Dr. DiMaria said, "and how lucky I am to be alive."

Virginia mother and kidney transplant recipient Amanda Bisnauth-Thomas was able to meet her donor's family, too, though in this case a whole gang of people had been saved.

Amanda had developed unexplained kidney failure that had become a life-threatening condition. Eventually, after an agonizing wait, Amanda received the kidney of a teenager, nineteen-year-old Jami Interiano, who had been a gunshot victim. After the donation, Jami's family wanted to meet his organ recipients. The day Amanda met Jami's family, she also met the patients who received Jami's other organs: Chuck Campbell, a car salesman from Delaware, who had received Jami's lungs; George Ortega, a limo driver from Florida, who had received his heart; and Kelly Coles, a nurse from Upper Marlboro, Maryland, who had received his other kidney. Together, they learned about the teenager who had saved their lives—a Dallas Cowboys fan who loved '80s music.

As reported in *Arlington Magazine* in December 2015, Amanda still maintains a relationship with the other organ recipients, especially Kelly Coles, the recipient of Jami's other kidney. They refer to each other as "kidney sisters." Jami's family now sees Amanda as one of their own, and Amanda reports with a laugh that she is "expected to take sides in family arguments."

I loved hearing about what transplants could do for people,

but I couldn't help but also wonder where it left families like ours. There was no mechanism in place to track results of donations that go to research rather than for transplant. It was clear from the outset that I might never be able to know for sure what became of Thomas's donation.

So I studied the outcome letters we had received from the various organizations.

The first one was a handwritten note from Heidi Cope at Duke, thanking us for participating in the anencephaly study. It was dated March 25, four days before Thomas died.

The next came from WRTC on April 6, a week after Thomas's funeral:

> Your son's liver was not able to be transplanted, but we are pleased to tell you that it was recovered for medical research, and will be included in a study on liver cell preparation for the treatment of severe metabolic disorders in newborn children.
>
> The intention of the study is to confirm that liver cell preparation can replace the missing enzymatic activity in the liver, which often results in self-intoxication of the body, lifelong brain dysfunction with mental retardation, and early death of newborn children.
>
> This medical study will use your loved one's liver cells to raise the enzymatic activity in the liver of the sick child until they have gained sufficient body weight to undergo a donor liver transplantation procedure, which can take place at the age of 12 to 18 weeks. Thank you for this invaluable contribution to this important research.
>
> Your son's corneas were unable to be transplanted; however, we are pleased to tell you that they were recov-

ered by Old Dominion Eye Foundation and provided
to National Development and Research Institutes, Inc.
for a very special education research project.

Old Dominion Eye Foundation was one of the oldest and
most respected eye banks in the country. Whereas OPOs like
WRTC perform organ and tissue recoveries, eye banking staff
sometimes perform the eye recovery and work alongside the
OPO professionals in the operating room.

When I looked up National Development and Research
Institutes, mentioned at the end of that letter, I didn't understand the connection, and a Google search initially didn't make
things clearer.

It turns out that that was because it was a typo: the organization is actually called the National *Disease* Research *Interchange,* and it serves as basically the Match.com of donation,
connecting available diseased and healthy tissue for research
with the researchers that need it. NDRI was founded in 1980
by a woman named Lee Ducat, whose son was diabetic. She
had wanted to help scientists studying diabetes find a cure,
and found out that what they needed were human pancreases.
Researchers had been finding their own from local hospitals
up to that point, but NDRI established a national network of
sources to provide pancreases so that researchers could focus
on their work instead of focusing on the often-fruitless search.
When scientists investigating other diseases learned of NDRI's
work, they started asking the organization to help them with
their tissue needs as well.

What started as Ducat's dream has transformed into a major
resource for the scientific community. (She turned NDRI over
in 2012 to Bill Leinweber, who came to the organization with
more than twenty-five years' experience advocating for medical

research.) NDRI now offers a catalogue of more than seven thousand biological specimens—collected from donors from more than 160 organ-procurement organizations, tissue banks, eye banks, and hospitals—and distributes nearly thirty thousand specimens annually to over five hundred academic, pharmaceutical, biotech, and medical-device organizations.

Donors don't even have to be deceased. NDRI also facilitates donations of tissue from surgery, such as tumors, or diseased organs such as lungs and livers that have been replaced with transplants.

The next week, I received two more letters. The first was forwarded to me from Immanuel Rasool, the manager of Research Donations at WRTC, who had received it from Cytonet in Durham, North Carolina.

> Please extend our gratitude and condolences to the family of your donor, a baby boy, for their willingness to give someone else the Gift of Life through research.
>
> Also, please thank your staff for everything they did to provide the opportunity of liver research to the baby's family.
>
> The process gave us a viability of 52.2% with 12.94 billion cells counted. The cells were not of the best quality and the viability was borderline. There were areas noted on the liver of pooled blood that looked like bruising. The remaining tissue was utilized in our lab for additional testing and research to assist in developing a better outcome for future cases.
>
> Once again, thank you to everyone involved at WRTC and the hospital and especially the family of this precious baby boy.

The next letter, from Old Dominion Eye Foundation, didn't include any additional information, just a sincere thank you and some grief materials. And the next, from WRTC in May, included a butterfly pin as a token of appreciation and remembrance.

And that was it. No more information, no more updates about what my son was doing, about whether his donations were having or would have an impact. So I did what I guess I was expected to do.

I got on with living.

Callum was an easy baby: he started sleeping through the night as soon as I went back to work. I think Ross and I were more laid-back than many first-time parents, perhaps because of what we'd gone through in the pregnancy. Problems that our fellow parents complained about—the cost and scarcity of quality day care, breast-feeding, pediatrician appointments, and nap schedules—didn't even register as real issues to us. We had a beautiful, healthy child with a completely formed skull. We were freaking delighted.

One of the things we worked hard at doing was maintaining our pre-baby lifestyle as much as possible while simply easing Callum into it. So, we brought him with us when we went out to dinner or traveled; by the time he was two years old, he had flown across the Atlantic and back three times to visit Ross's family in Scotland. Ross still played on his rugby team and went to the pub at seven o'clock in the morning to watch Glasgow Celtic and the Scottish national soccer team. I picked up my graduate school studies at American University; I had four classes to go to get my master's degree in public communications.

In one class, we had been asked to give a presentation about the challenges of surveys; I did mine on my experience of filling out the survey for the Duke anencephaly study. Using PowerPoint slides that included photos of Thomas and Callum, I explained to the class what had made me a motivated participant (it meant my child's death was not in vain) and where the pitfalls had been (embarrassing questions; the burden of things like getting blood draws; needing favors from busy medical staff). It turned out the exercise of making my experience the subject of a presentation was therapeutic; it was the first time I was able to discuss what had happened at a remove. It was starting, very slowly, to become a piece of my history rather than as something I was going through every minute of every day.

During those first few months, I made the mistake of thinking that because the worst thing had already happened—my child had died—I was immune from anything bad happening again, at least for a while. But life doesn't work like that.

When my favorite coworker announced she was leaving her job, I went home and cried. I guess that from the outside it might not seem like a big deal, but it felt enormous to me at the time. When I pulled myself together, I realized that life would continue to throw me curveballs. Life was not singling me out for the bad, or the good. It was just life. I remembered some passages from *When Bad Things Happen to Good People*. Mother Teresa, one of the nicest people I could think of, still had bad things happen to her. Being nice, or having one terrible thing happen to you, doesn't provide an invisible force field that shields you from the normal ups and downs of life. You can't control things that way.

My family was devastated when my stepfather, Bob, unexpectedly died of a heart attack in December 2010, only nine months after Thomas passed away. We're not a very religious family, and we didn't belong to a church, so we asked Phil

Brooks to perform the service, and Bob was buried in the same cemetery as Thomas.

As we approached the one-year anniversary of Thomas's death, I found myself caring more and more about what had happened with his donations. I decided to contact Old Dominion Eye Foundation to see if they had any follow-up information, so I sent them an email. I got the following response:

——————Forwarded message——————
From: Christina Jenkins
Date: Wed, Feb 9, 2011 at 12:56 PM
Subject: RE: Contact Request From ODEF Website
To: Sarah Gray

Ms. Gray,

Thomas' donated eyes were used as part of research program at the Schepens Eye Research Institute. . . . [Schepens is] involved in many valuable research studies conquering diseases of the eye. We all know someone who has been touched with these debilitating diseases. Please take comfort in knowing that countless individuals are being helped with his donation and that their renewed vision is a legacy left by your son. I offer my deepest sympathies as you approach the one-year anniversary of Thomas' passing.

Sincerely,

Christina Jenkins

Once I'd finished reading the note, I Googled "Schepens," and was delighted to see that the institute was part of Harvard Medical School.

Thomas Ethan Gray had gotten into Harvard.

On the first anniversary of Thomas's death, we visited his grave. When we buried him a year earlier, his small plot had been on the outer row of this small cluster of lost babies. Because his tombstone was not ready at the time, a brass stake with a typed paper sign had designated his space. He had been the newest addition to his row.

Now, a year later, his permanent tombstone was in place, and the grass had grown over some, but newer graves surrounded his, each with a new brass stake. For some reason, I expected that Thomas's grave would be the last. It still seemed so recent to me. How is it that so many more babies had died since last year?

Ross and I touched Thomas's tombstone, brushed off the dust, and left him some flowers. A breeze made the chimes in the nearby trees sound softly, as though to acknowledge our presence. With the tinkling sound all around us, we turned and walked away.

A few weeks later, we attended WRTC's annual donor-family gathering, which is held every spring in memory of those who have "given the gift of life."

We had been invited to contribute a square to the annual WRTC donor quilt. The tradition had begun in 1995 as a memorial to donors. The quilts hang in the WRTC offices, but they also travel to community meetings, health fairs, press conferences, and informational presentations around Washington, DC, Maryland, and Virginia. Thomas's quilt was the fifteenth such quilt, and it would be unveiled at a service at the National Presbyterian Church in Washington, DC. His square comprised several photos of Thomas and Callum and one photo of Thomas solo, Ross's left hand covering his tiny chest. (Revered newsman Tim Russert, who died suddenly of a heart attack in 2008, was also a donor, and has a square on WRTC's thirteenth quilt. His gave a shout-out to his beloved Buffalo Bills and to *Meet the Press,* the program he'd moderated on NBC for many years.) The gathering was attended by donor families, recipients, transplant surgeons, WRTC staff, and other people from the transplant community, and was followed by a lovely reception.

I was especially moved by a poem that was written and delivered by Dr. James Selby Jr., a heart and two-time kidney recipient. It was a poem called "You," and it was dedicated to his organ donor. It began with the words:

> *I remember when I first found out,*
> *that my organs were coming from you.*
> *A sense of happiness filled my heart,*
> *however there was a feeling of sadness too.*
> *For me to live,*
> *you had to die.*
> *While my family rejoiced,*
> *your family cried.*

I thought about the researchers who received Thomas's organs.

Just as so many people are touched by the gift of an organ for transplant, I figured someone out there must have been touched by Thomas's donation for research. Who received the package with Thomas's liver? Did they wonder about him or his family? Is it weird to open a package that contains the eyes of a fellow member of the human race? How many packages do they open per year, or per day? Was there a crowd of eye researchers rejoicing with its arrival? Or was it stored on a shelf, collecting dust?

Although the counseling had been helpful, it wasn't the only thing I needed. I was looking for some kind of peace. I thought that perhaps I should try a psychic; I don't believe in them, but I was curious, and wanted something or someone to give me perspective on my loss.

My sister-in-law Julia went to a psychic called Kizzy, in Glasgow, in 2012. Julia reported in an email that Kizzy had told her that Thomas was "at peace and with his own people and was looking after his wee bro," that Thomas "had to go to let Callum live and he knew from the beginning that he didn't have long. . . . He waited to meet the family and make sure Callum was OK and he was at peace when he died with all his family around him."

On the second anniversary of the twins' birth, I sent an update to the twins' medical team, with a photo of Callum and a précis of what the psychic had said. Phil Brooks wrote back:

> In your last email you had mentioned what a psychic
> had said . . . and I had a similar experience but have hes-
> itated to share it with you. Maybe a phone chat would
> be better.

By total coincidence, Phil—a spiritually open-minded person—occasionally speaks to a psychic named Claudia Coronado in Sedona, Arizona, to "get clarity on issues." It just so happened, he told me, that in a meeting with her in September 2009, when I was pregnant, she told him that "there were two souls waiting to enter the world that I [i.e., Phil] would be deeply involved with. She indicated they were looking forward to meeting me, but there was one who was going to need me especially." Phil had no idea what she was referring to, not even when he met us at the twins' birth.

I was so grateful for the care I had received from the hospital staff, including my doctors, some nurses, and the chaplain, that I wrote a letter to the hospital CEO, and recognized each person for his or her contribution. As a result, these hospital employees were selected to receive an Inova Service Legends Award.

When Callum was six months old, we attended the awards ceremony. Phil asked if he could hold Callum, who had been fussing. As soon as Phil picked him up, Callum looked into his eyes and put his head on Phil's shoulder. He didn't do that with anyone else. Phil said to him, "Do you remember me?" Callum lifted his head up and looked into Phil's eyes again, then put his head back down on his shoulder. Phil thought, *I believe that some part of him knows me.* And it was then that he remembered his conversation with Claudia the psychic, though it would take him some time to tell us about it.

On the second anniversary of Thomas's death, in March 2012, I called Claudia Coronado for a reading of my own. When I asked Claudia what she charged, she said she didn't because she couldn't guarantee that she'd be able to contact the right people.

"Thomas has appeared to you before, right?" Claudia said.

I told her he hadn't.

"He's a golden light," she said, as though I had answered in the affirmative. "He will appear to his brother. If his brother says he's talked to him, believe him."

I nodded into the phone and let her continue.

"Thomas's role now is like a teacher; he helps people who have just come to the other side. He welcomes them and makes them feel comfortable and makes sure that they know that everything is okay there."

Even though it sounded like a bunch of baloney, I still found it comforting to picture him in this role. I guess I wanted it to be true.

"He will also make sure that your family is okay financially."

The lottery ticket I wrote to him about?

"You'll be having another baby, a girl. And I see the girl bringing a boy with her."

Claudia asked me if there was anyone else I might like to learn about.

I told her my stepfather had died just a few months earlier.

"I see him. He's saying, 'But . . . but . . . but . . . that's it?' He is struggling to accept his fate."

She said that Thomas was there to calm people like my stepfather who were unsettled by their own death.

"Your mother will get married again to a nice man."

(Three years later, she would do so, but when Claudia made this prediction, my mother hadn't even met him.)

Whether any of it was true or not, the way Claudia described Thomas made me imagine him as a mature adult with a job. Even more, it made me think he was in the right place, especially when his time on earth hadn't seemed to suit him at all.

During a visit to see Ross's family in March 2013, I decided to go see the psychic Kizzy for myself. I had been warned that she was so popular people lined up to see her and that the doors opened at 8 A.M., so I made sure to arrive by 7 A.M. so I would be first in line. Her "office" was on the top floor of a dilapidated shopping center called the Savoy Centre, on Argyle Street in Glasgow.

At 7 A.M. the metal grate was still down on the shop door, so I stood outside reading *The Immortal Life of Henrietta Lacks,* by Rebecca Skloot. I was enthralled by the story of this woman whose cancerous cells had led to so many remarkable advancements in medical science, albeit without her or her family's consent or knowledge.

Every few minutes, more people—mostly young and middle-aged women—collected in the line behind me.

"Here to see Kizzy?" we asked one another.

By 8 A.M. there were about twenty people in line behind me, and Kizzy's "handler" appeared. He counted from one to fifteen, and told the people from sixteen on to come back another day because she would not have time to see them before 4 P.M., when she saw her last customer.

He told the people from number ten to fifteen that she might not be able to see them, either, because "she can take twenty minutes, or she can take an hour. It's whatever she's feeling." They all agreed to wait.

"We drove down from Aberdeen to see her," I heard someone say. Aberdeen is a three-hour drive from Glasgow on a good day.

Four people showed the handler their "jump the line" cards, which they were given because they had previously waited an entire day and had not been able to see Kizzy before she closed. These four were let in ahead of me.

When the mall opened, the metal grate rolled up and we were led to her office. The mall was dark, seedy, outdated. One shop sold tacky nightclub wear along with light bulbs, First Communion dresses, and sympathy cards. Another seemed to provide an unlocking service for stolen cell phones. I was hungry for coffee and a bagel or toast, but before I could get something, the handler told me it was my turn.

Kizzy didn't look like the stereotypical psychic, with the earrings and crystal ball. She had graying black hair and was wearing the sensible clothing of a normal sixty-something-year-old woman. She looked like my mom, and when she spoke she had a slight Eastern European accent.

As soon as I sat down and introduced myself, Kizzy touched my wrist and said, "I just got a warm feeling shooting up my arm. I am feeling a presence."

She went on to tell me that the presence was Thomas.

"I see you at your job; you wear a name badge."

I did, but so did lots of people.

"Your grandfather was in the war."

Wasn't everybody's grandfather in one war or another?

Then she said, "I see you at a book signing."

A lot of people had told me to write a book. This was starting to freak me out.

The book thing gave me a weird sensation; it was too much.
I felt dizzy. Even though it was not yet 10 A.M., it made me
want to get a stiff drink—or go on a trip, far away from my
regular routine.

I was also afraid. Did I believe her? Am I the kind of person
who believes psychics now? I was scared to believe her. But if I
didn't believe her, why had I just waited three hours in line and
paid her? What was I even doing here?

I didn't believe everything she said, but I have spent forty
pounds sterling in worse ways.

When I returned home, I was different. It was time to do
something.

CHAPTER SEVEN

An Accidental Quest Begins—
Schepens Eye Research Institute
July 31, 2012

I n late July 2012, I was scheduled to take a business trip to
Boston, and I invited my mom to join me with the intention of squeezing in a couple of fun dinners and maybe
some sightseeing in between my work obligations.

In the week leading up to the trip, I did some research
about Schepens Eye Research Institute, which I discovered was
less than two miles from the John B. Hynes Veterans Memorial
Convention Center, where I'd be working during the day.

The institute was founded in 1950 as the Retina Foundation by Charles L. Schepens, who would become known as the
father of modern retinal surgery. Schepens, a Belgian national
who fled his country when it was overrun by the Germans
in 1940, spent much of the war working with the French and
Belgian resistance, and was arrested by the Gestapo more than
once. He eventually found his way to London, where he began
working as a retinal surgeon. After the war, he emigrated to the
United States and took a position at the ophthalmology lab at

Harvard Medical School. Just two years later, he founded the world's first medical practice for treating diseases and conditions of the retina, at Massachusetts Eye and Ear Infirmary. Over the course of his long and accomplished career, Dr. Schepens developed numerous ophthalmic instruments and pioneered many surgical procedures, all of which, when combined, are credited with more than doubling the success rate of retinal reattachment surgery from 40 percent to 90 percent.

Today's Schepens Eye Research Institute—it joined forces with Massachusetts Eye and Ear in 2011 and is an affiliate of Harvard Medical School—is one of the leading eye-research institutions in the country. Its mission is to find new ways to treat and cure eye disorders. Since its inception, its work has expanded to include such cutting-edge innovations as gene therapy, stem-cell research, nerve regeneration, and tissue engineering—all in hopes of finding cures and treatments for the leading causes of blindness and vision impairment.

I combed the Schepens website to see if I could figure out which scientist or study might have received Thomas's donation. I hoped that I could make a connection with someone who could give me a tour while I was in town. I found email addresses for a couple of scientists there, and sent them each a message explaining who I was and asking to arrange a visit.

A volunteer patient liaison wrote back to me to say that because of privacy restrictions, he would not be able to tell me how, or even *if,* my son's donation was used. He made no mention of my request for a tour. So I set out for Boston with no visit to Schepens planned. I hoped I might hear from one of the people I'd emailed before I arrived, but no such luck.

A few days into my trip, I decided to give it one last shot, and a Google search produced the phone number of the Schepens front desk. For a second I was shocked to realize the place had a front desk. If I was willing to make one of the weirdest calls of my life, maybe something would happen.

I paced the skywalk of the Hynes Convention Center as I imagined how the call might go. I would explain the whole story and they would tell me it violated some confidentiality thing. Or that it wasn't allowed. Or it wasn't within policy. But I thought, *I have a personal connection to this place. I gave them something they needed. I'm sure they have wondered, at some point, where the donations came from. I'm just going to call. I will feel awkward. Maybe they'll feel awkward, too. If I could just get past the part of talking about the death of a child to a complete stranger over the phone, something powerful might happen. I have to at least try.*

My heart raced as I clicked "Dial," and I gripped the phone hard.

Here goes. I am doing this.

"Schepens Eye Research Institute. How can I help you?" a woman's voice said.

Adrenaline shot through me. I tried to play it cool: Shucks, I'm just a regular old girl next door looking for her deceased child's cornea researcher. Just like everybody else.

"Hi, my name is Sarah Gray. I have a kind of unusual request, but maybe you can point me in the right direction." I could feel my face get hot. "I had an infant son who died of a birth defect a few years ago. And we donated his eyes to Schepens." My heart was thumping hard now. "I live in Washington, DC, but I am here in Boston on business for the next few days, and I was wondering if I could get, like, a ten-minute tour while I am in town—just so I can learn more about what Schepens does."

There was a long pause, and then the woman changed everything. She said, "I've never had a request like this, but I will find someone to help you. Please stay on the line, okay? It might take a while, but I'll find someone."

I was expecting to hang up in tears, but my hopes soared. Was this actually going to work?

After a while, I was put through to Carolyn Bellefeuille in the development department.

"I'm so sorry to hear about your son. Twins, was it?" She had a New England accent.

"Yes. His brother is fine, a very healthy little boy."

"My daughter just had twins. They were born premature—thirty-three and a half weeks—but now they're fine. How old is your boy?"

"He's two."

"So this is a big facility, and there is a lot to see. Do you know which part you are interested in seeing? Retina? Cornea?"

The letter I'd received from WRTC had mentioned Thomas's eyes, but nothing more specific. "Wherever you think my son's eyes would have gone," I said. "Do you have a place for pediatric eyes?"

"No, but we have areas for cornea research and retina research. I'm sorry to ask this, but it might help if you can tell me how he died."

"Technically, his heart stopped, but he had anencephaly. Part of his brain was missing."

"In that case, he probably donated corneas, not retinas. I can show you the area where they do the cornea research."

It was refreshing to talk to a stranger about Thomas in a new context rather than through the lens of grief. Carolyn and I were talking about Thomas's eye donation, a topic about as uncomfortable and unusual as you can get, but it didn't feel that way. There was no pity in her voice. She agreed to meet my mom and me at noon the next day.

Something inside me started to shift.

When we pulled up in front of the unassuming red brick building in West Boston the next day, I saw the Schepens logo by the door, and my heart jumped. I started making a mental list of the photos I wanted to take to share with Ross and Callum.

I noticed a FedEx delivery truck near the loading dock, and I wondered if it was delivering eye tissue to the scientists. I wondered if Thomas's donation had come in through this loading dock, too.

Once inside, I was in awe. I felt like I was in Santa's workshop. I read the names of the financial benefactors on the wall and felt like one of them, even though my name wasn't listed. This place was now part of my permanent family history. As I looked around the lobby, Thomas stopped being just a memory. He had an address in the real world. I could take a taxi to an actual place *where he was.* There were secretaries working there and microwaving Lean Cuisines for lunch. This place had a website and brochures; in fact, I took one about eye care and stuffed it into my purse, just to prove that this was not a dream.

"So nice to meet you," Carolyn said when she came to greet us, reaching for my hand to shake it. She was an older woman with dark black hair and kind green eyes. "We have never had a donor's family here before."

And so began the tour. Carolyn walked us through several labs, where we saw people in their twenties and thirties hunched over microscopes. She explained that most of the research was done with animals on the lower level, but we were not allowed to go down there because of the sterile environment. We saw refrigerators and freezers and microwaves with "No Food" signs taped on them, and another handwritten sign that read something like "Please do not mix mammalian cells."

Eventually we reached the desk of a man eating a salad from Whole Foods. It was Dr. James Zieske, a senior scientist at

Schepens and an associate professor of ophthalmology at Harvard Medical School. He had grayish brown hair, round cheeks, large wire-frame glasses, and a friendly smile. I would learn later that Dr. Zieske had been studying the mechanisms involved in repairing wounds to the cornea for thirty years and had published more than seventy peer-reviewed articles on the subject. Incredibly, he was also the man who ordered the human eyes for research. In other words, he was one of the people I had been wondering about for the last two years.

When Carolyn explained who we were, Dr. Zieske looked shaken. He immediately stood up from his desk and shook our hands.

"Thank you so much for your donation. We can't do our work without such gifts." He paused. "Do you have any questions for me?"

I struggled to catch my breath to speak. I was afraid that the questions I wanted to ask would seem morbid or would break some rule of confidentiality. But I knew I might never get this chance again. The atmosphere was so charged, it was glimmering.

I said, "How do you order eyes? Is there a catalog?"

"Yes, actually, there is. We order them online from an eye bank."

"How do the eyes arrive? Do they come in the mail? Or FedEx?"

"They are shipped FedEx, and they arrive over in that mail room." He pointed to a doorway in the back of the lab.

"How many eyes do you order in a year?"

"My department orders about ten pairs per year. But the facility, as a whole, orders about a hundred pairs a year. We would order more if we could, but they are hard to get. That's why most of the research is done on animal eyes first. When the backup research is done, then we move on to study human eyes."

I pulled up a photo on my phone of the twins, and I zoomed in on Thomas's eyes. "Here is a picture of my son. Do you remember getting these eyes?" They seemed like a unique pair of eyes to me. One of his eyes had been swollen, round, and pink and about the size of a large gumball, and the other was the size of a jellybean.

Dr. Zieske smiled kindly at me. "By the time we get them, the eyes have been processed. We only get the corneas, and they all look the same. Kind of like contact lenses. But most of the eyes we get are from older people. Infant eyes are like gold to us."

I choked down a sob.

"Why do you say that?"

"Young tissue has a much greater potential to regenerate. If you don't mind me asking, when did your son die?"

"About two years ago."

"The tissue can regenerate for up to two years, so we are probably still using his eye cells right now."

I was stunned. The donation was so much more valuable than I had even dared imagine.

Dr. Zieske went on to explain that there are three types of cells in the cornea: the epithelium, the stromal fibroblasts, and the endothelium. Both the epithelium and fibroblasts proliferate both in the cornea and in culture, but the endothelial cells do not proliferate in the cornea after birth. So the cells you are born with are the only ones you get. In a culture, the endothelial cells can be coaxed into proliferating, although it is a tricky process. The scientist who actually received Thomas's cornea was one of the leaders, before she retired, in developing methods to get endothelial cells to proliferate. Her process is now widely used as a source of cells that can be transplanted into eyes in which the endothelial cell number has dropped to an unhealthy level.

I savored every second in Dr. Zieske's presence. It felt so important and special to be there, like I was meeting Bruce Springsteen or an astronaut or a *Titanic* survivor. I asked him questions just to have a reason to be in his presence longer. I felt a love for him the way I love my brothers. I pictured us being friends. I pictured Ross and me being invited to his house for a dinner party.

This was a landmark day in my life, and I wanted to record it. So I asked my mom to take my picture with Dr. Zieske and Carolyn.

Eventually we had to say good-bye to Dr. Zieske—I wanted to let him finish his lunch—and Carolyn led us to the elevator, where we passed a young man with brown hair and a Russian accent talking to a colleague in the hallway. Carolyn whispered, "That's probably one of the smartest people in the world. He is doing groundbreaking work with retinas."

I believed her. This seemed like a place where The Smartest Person in the World might actually hang out.

Next stop was the office of Dr. Andrius Kazlauskas, a macular regeneration specialist and Harvard Medical School professor. He had short, white hair and a trimmed beard, and there was a bicycle in his office. Dr. Kaslauskas was kind, though he seemed a little unsure of what to say. He told us that he was researching retinopathy in premature babies (a condition that can lead to permanent blindness), and he asked what else I might like to know.

"I've met a lot of people who got the chance to meet their donor's recipient and shake their hands," I said, starting to melt with tears. "But since I donated my son's organs to research rather than for transplant, I don't know what happened to the donations. So that's why I'm here. I just want to learn what happens in a place like this. And I am really impressed and glad we were able to donate here."

Dr. Kaslauskas put his arm around me as my mom took another picture. My smile was ugly because I was still crying.

Next on the tour, Carolyn showed us a six-hundred-thousand-dollar microscope called a confocal that was probably used to look at my son's eye cells. It was enormous, and had not only its own room but its own staff member, Dr. Donald Pottle, who guarded it. I noticed that there were photos of eyes decorating the walls, and Dr. Pottle laughed and said these were pictures of his own eyes he had taken for fun.

Carolyn then took us through the area where blind people could simulate driving a car, and areas where experiments are conducted to see how eyes behave and what kinds of things they focus on. She showed us a picture on the wall of another doctor, Tatsuo Hirose; she said he has "magic hands" and has restored vision in many babies. He was wearing the classic white lab coat, with wire-rimmed spectacles on his round face and a sweet, kind smile on his lips. I took a photo of his photo.

It seemed like a place where anything can happen, where the smartest people from all over the world meet to solve real problems. It refreshed my spirit to be in this positive place filled with positive people doing positive things.

All too soon the visit was over. Carolyn said she could tell that the doctors were moved by my visit, and we agreed to keep in touch.

As we were leaving, she said, "I will never forget you."

Back at the convention center, I felt myself floating, watching everything as if from above. My mind was still at Schepens.

I was grateful that my mom had been with me for such a special occasion. Thomas was hers, too, not just mine. And I was glad to have a witness to prove that it wasn't just a dream.

That night, my mom and I talked as we lay in our beds with the lights out.

"I still can't believe I set that up," I said. "I didn't think they would let me in. And I didn't know much I needed that until it happened. I feel a sense of peace."

The Hail Mary pass I had thrown into the universe had been caught. I now had a new way to think of my son. He has a job. He has coworkers. He has colleagues. He is a partner in their research, and relevant in this community. They cannot do their job without him.

The next day, my mom bought a toddler-size Harvard T-shirt for Callum that featured the Harvard school motto: *Veritas.*

Truth.

The whole experience at Schepens had been a revelation to me, but apparently I had been something of a revelation to them as well. A few days later, I received an email:

Dear Mrs. Gray,

Thank you for the kind words and the pictures. I'm glad that we could reassure you that your donation did make a difference.

When we get eyes from the Eye Bank, they are provided to us with minimal identifying information as required by law. We are told the age, sex, and cause of death. When we are offered young eyes like your son's, we are pleased because we know that young tissue has much more potential to grow than older tissue. We tend to not dwell on the source of the eyes. Your visit helped to remind me that all the eyes we receive are an incredibly generous gift from someone who loved and cared about the person who provided the eyes. I thank you for reminding me of this.

Sincerely,

Jim Zieske

CHAPTER EIGHT

The Quest Continues—Duke

*A Tour of the Anencephaly Study at Duke
University Medical Center*
November 11, 2012

The experience of visiting Schepens had been so powerful that I asked myself, *Can I do this at the other facilities, too?* I wanted to at least try to visit the places that received Thomas's liver and cord blood.

I called Maureen Balderston, a donor-family advocate at WRTC, and told her about my Boston adventure. She sounded a little shocked, maybe even a bit scared. Clearly what I had done wasn't common.

"In fifteen years, I have never heard of anyone doing this," Maureen said. "Was it a good experience?"

"It was an amazing experience," I said, "and I want keep going. Can you arrange a meeting for me at Cytonet, the place that received Thomas's liver? I'm going to call the folks at the Duke and see if I can get a tour there, too. Since they're both located in Durham, I could visit them on the same trip."

"I'll see what I can do," she said.

In the meantime, I emailed Heidi Cope at Duke to ask if I could bring my family by for a tour.

I wanted Ross and Callum to join me for the road trip to Durham. I wanted Ross to experience the healing that I felt during the visit to Schepens. I knew that as the years went on, the people who were involved in Thomas's donation might no longer work there. And if I wanted to meet the people who were actually involved, the sooner we did it, the better.

"I know what a lab looks like," Ross said. "It's not going to bring him back."

"Why not go? We've never been to Durham. It's only a five-hour drive. We can go the night before, stay downtown, and explore the city. Maybe there's a sports thing there."

This made the difference, since Ross is always up for exploring new places, especially places with sports teams and stadiums he can spot. He's like a bird-watcher, but with stadiums, and the prospect of visiting the home of the Durham Bulls sealed the deal.

We arrived in Durham the evening of Sunday, November 10, 2012. After checking in to the downtown Marriott, we walked through City Center Plaza, home to the imposing bronze Durham Bull statue, then headed to a local microbrewery for dinner. While two-and-a-half-year-old Callum played with a pile of toys, and Ross and I enjoyed an after-dinner beer, I thought, *How did we wind up taking this trip?* We were being pulled in a direction by our son who was no longer with us. Thomas was the reason we were there.

It felt like we were on a mission.

The next morning, we drove to the Snyderman Building at Duke University Medical Center, which housed the Duke anencephaly study. The genetic researchers who were located in the Snyderman Building studied a wide range of conditions but were united by their efforts to understand the "genetic basis of human disease." The ten or so faculty members were involved in more than three hundred studies, including the mapping or identification of genes in more than fifty diseases, including Alzheimer's, heart disease, glaucoma, autism, Parkinson's, macular degeneration, muscular dystrophy, and multiple sclerosis.

Though we would be meeting with researchers from the Duke anencephaly study, these researchers were investigating not just anencephaly but cardiovascular disease, liver disease, muscular and neurodegenerative disorders, psychiatric disorders, and even cancer. They believe that their work on multiple conditions makes them better scientists because what they learn from one condition can help them better understand other conditions.

As we approached the Duke University campus, I felt my heart pound. It was like we were visiting Thomas at college. I thought, *This must be what it was like for my parents to visit me years earlier in a strange town that was not their home.* Now Thomas was introducing us to new places, new people, and new ideas.

Once again I imagined a FedEx package, with Thomas's and Callum's blood this time, being delivered to the front desk. I took a picture of Ross outside the building, crouched down next to Callum's stroller.

On our arrival, Heidi Cope, a blond woman with big blue eyes, greeted us. It was Heidi with whom I'd spoken on the phone more than two years earlier. She brought us upstairs to a large, glass-walled conference room, where we were joined by a group of researchers. Heidi's job was to handle enrollment of participants in the study. Allison Ashley-Koch, Ph.D., a genetic epidemiologist, focuses on the genetic, epigenetic (more on this in a minute), and environmental contributions to neural tube defects—and also just happens to be a codirector of the largest

genetic study of anencephaly in the world. Dr. Simon Gregory is the other codirector; he works on genomics and epigenetics, too, and is also the director of the genomic laboratory
at the David H. Murdock Research Institute. Dr. Gregory, who
had brown hair, wire-frame glasses, and an Australian accent,
had previously led the effort to map the mouse genome and to
sequence human chromosome 1 for the Human Genome Project. Deidre Krupp, who also attended the meeting, was a graduate student under Dr. Gregory and had worked most closely
with the twins' blood.

Dr. Gregory explained that having access to the cord blood
of a set of identical twins who were "discordant"—one was
healthy and one had the fatal genetic defect—was incredibly
valuable. Since identical twins are genetically the same and their
in utero environment is the same—same mom, same placenta,
same amount of folic acid—Thomas and Callum provided an
unusual opportunity to investigate what else might have caused
the discrepancy in their development.

As for the anencephaly study that we took part in, the
researchers looked specifically at a kind of epigenetics called
DNA methylation. Although identical twins have identical
genes, their epigenetic process—the process by which genes get
turned on and off—can be different. If DNA is the "hardware,"
the DNA methylation and the epigenetic changes are the "software."

These kinds of changes are easily caused by environmental factors and can have a significant impact on the expression
of genes. It is known, for instance, that maternal smoking can
change the methylation in particular regions of the genome in
utero, although that wasn't relevant to Thomas since I didn't
smoke. And these changes are also different from cell type to
cell type: a change in the blood will be different from changes

in the liver or brain; even within the brain, there are different cell types, so the changes will vary within the brain itself.

Folic acid, like smoking, can also affect epigenetics, which is why, starting in 1991, the Centers for Disease Control and Prevention has recommended that women trying to get pregnant take four hundred micrograms of it every day. A year later, the U.S. Public Health Service recommended that all women of childbearing age take folic acid, since about half of all pregnancies are unplanned, and neural tube defects occur so early in a pregnancy that by the time a woman knows she's pregnant it's too late to begin supplementation. By the mid-1990s, the U.S. government was mandating folic acid fortification in cereal grain products such as bread. As a result, the number of neural tube defects began to drop dramatically.

However, the fact that these defects still occur suggests either that some mothers aren't able to process folic acid, in which case it wouldn't matter how much they took; that some mothers are susceptible to too much folic acid; or that there was something else in the environment causing the defect.

Deidre Krupp, the graduate student, told us that she had presented a poster based on some discoveries from a small sample, including what might be the twins' blood samples, at a conference. Professionals who discover something interesting or want to present their findings to their professional peers create a poster to display at a conference, like a science-fair project for grown-ups.

"You made a poster? Do you still have it? Can I see it?" I was astounded and excited.

Deidre went to fetch the poster. It was an aqua-green poster with the title "Genetic and Epigenetic Variances in Twins Discordant for Anencephaly." The eight authors (Deidre Krupp, Christina A. Markunas, Karen Soldano, Kaia S. Quinn, Heidi

Cope, Melanie E. Garrett, Allison E. Ashley-Koch, and Simon G. Gregory) laid out in two columns their research into "a mono-zygotic twin pair discordant for anencephaly." The whole thing was dense with scientific jargon, so I went straight to the con-clusion: "findings support potential causative role for altered methylation in NTD (neural tube defects) etiology, particularly in concert with predisposing genetic variation."

"What does this mean?"

"There are epigenetic differences between the twins, and they seem to be random," Deidre said.

"Do you think this was caused by me using a sauna or being hot?"

"I could never rule that out, but no—based on what we saw, I don't think so."

"Were you surprised by this?"

Deidre laughed, then paused before saying, "No. Because for me to be surprised, that implies that I knew what to expect. We are only in the beginning stage of trying to understand what causes anencephaly."

Until that moment, I had often wondered what I might have done to cause Thomas's anencephaly. Now I was being told that the answers were not clear at all, which was somewhat comforting: there was a distinct possibility I had not done any-thing wrong.

Deidre and Dr. Gregory explained that the anencephaly was likely caused by epigenetic markers. Sometimes epigenetic markers are caused by environmental factors in our lives, and sometimes they are passed down from our ancestors. As just one example, the effects of your grandfather's polluted work envi-ronment, or poor nutrition, may be passed down to you. This was an incredible thing to learn, and meant that the true causes of Thomas's condition might never be known.

In the acknowledgments sections of the poster the researchers had written:

The authors wish to thank the patients and family members for their participation in and contribution to this NTD study.

This was very poignant for me. We would never have known of the study or this acknowledgment if we hadn't decided to follow the trail of Thomas's donation. These twenty words were a thank-you letter that was never mailed—in fact, I wondered if the researchers were even *allowed* to contact us. In my dream world, we would have been emailed this study when it first came out.

Whatever the truth of the complicated nature of the relationship between research participants and scientists, something more important was true: there it was, proof of Thomas's contribution to science. Now I could finally celebrate the work I had done to provide decent blood samples. Just as the folks at the study were grateful for our donation, so I was grateful to Deidre and the team for taking the time to explain this important study to us.

This was part of Thomas's legacy, more work to which he had contributed. Maybe, thanks at least in part to him, babies of the future wouldn't suffer from the awful affliction that took his life. I was so proud of my son.

After we met the researchers, Karen Soldano, a lab research analyst, gave us a tour of the facility and showed us where the FedEx package of test tubes would have arrived, and where the blood was currently being stored (along with thousands of other samples). We saw rows of microscopes and equipment I had seen only on forensic science shows.

We were asked not to lean on the $150,000 DNA coding machine.

At the conclusion of the tour, we said our good-byes and hugged the researchers. Dr. Gregory thanked us for visiting, and told us that meeting us had reminded him of the personal investment in every blood sample they get.

We left with a new perspective on the complicated biological processes that result in human beings being born healthy—or not. Dr. Gregory had explained that they still couldn't tell us exactly what caused a defect or how to cure or prevent it—but it gave me great hope to know that the work they were doing could lead to clinically actionable information down the road. Maybe not for me, but for other people in the world who might one day be in my shoes.

This visit gave me a better appreciation for what researchers do, too. They face years of trial and error before they can ever point to a success. Dr. Gregory put it like this: "You have to be something of a masochist to be a scientist, because not every experiment works. It's 95 percent disappointment. We live for the 5 percent, when we are able to identify something no one has ever seen before." It occurred to me that scientists have something in common with organ, eye, and tissue donor families: we all do something to help people we may never meet.

We stopped off at the Duke University gift shop and got Callum another T-shirt.

CHAPTER NINE

The Quest Continues—Cytonet

A Tour of Cytonet, LLC
Later the Same Day

O ur next stop was Cytonet, the international biotech company that received Thomas's liver.

Cytonet is a for-profit, privately funded company. I imagined that Cytonet would have been founded or funded by someone with a personal connection to liver disease, but that was not the case.

The Cytonet Group was founded at the turn of the new millennium as a small spinoff from the cell-therapy division of the German biotech giant Roche Diagnostic GmbH, which itself was started in 1896 by Fritz Hoffmann-La Roche, an entrepreneur who believed that the mass production of medicine would be a major advance in treating disease.

Dr. Wolfgang Rüdinger, the physician who founded Cytonet, had been managing various programs within Roche, including a cell-therapy program. He realized he had a soft spot in his heart for treating patients with the lowest chance of survival and the fewest options, and had been working on developing a liver-cell therapy. When Roche decided to divest itself of its noncore assets, he left and took the technology with him to launch the new firm. Rüdinger joined forces with the investor Dietmar Hopp, a billionaire software expert who had recently resigned his position as co-CEO of the software behemoth SAP. Once an avid investor in such diverse holdings as breweries and sports teams, Hopp had since become an avid investor in biotech companies in Germany, in the hope of making his country a leader in the field. (Hopp's initial and continuing investment in Cytonet makes him its largest shareholder.)

In 2006, Cytonet partnered with, and ultimately took over various assets of, an American company called Vesta Therapeutics, Inc., based in Durham, North Carolina, giving them a toehold in the United States. Mark Johnston, a London Business School–trained entrepreneur who had been president of Vesta Therapeutics, became president and COO of Cytonet in 2009. Today Cytonet's staff of fifty is evenly divided between its Durham headquarters and its German location. Its focus is in the field of regenerative medicine, and its self-proclaimed mission is to "provide alternatives to existing therapies for many diseases with a particular emphasis on liver diseases."

When I first emailed Mark Johnston to follow up on the appointment that Maureen Balderston at WRTC had arranged, he graciously invited us to join him and his staff for lunch, in addition to the tour and presentation he was planning for us. And like others before him, he wanted to know what we wanted to know.

There was so much. I told him that in my fantasy world I'd love to see Thomas's liver cells under a microscope, but I knew that his cells were probably confidential, unidentifiable, and might not even still be there, so I'd be grateful to see *any* liver cells. Then I fired off a list of other things on my mind:

Who orders the liver samples, and when?

How do they decide when it's time to order a new one?

Where do the samples come from? The United States only, or all over the world?

What information is provided about the donor? Age, cause of death . . . ?

What happens after a sample arrives?

Who receives it, and where does it go next?

How many scientists use one sample?

How long is one sample typically used until it's used up? How long does one sample last?

How many samples are ordered in a normal year?

Has there ever been a sample shortage (a backorder situation)?

When we arrived at Cytonet's headquarters, located in an unassuming office park, Mark Johnston was there to greet us. Mark looked to be in his forties, had a close-cropped beard and hair, and was wearing a sharp blue suit. "We are really glad you came," he said. And like others before him elsewhere, he commented that this was the first-ever donor visit.

Mark introduced us to several members of the Cytonet staff—Sonya Meheux, manager of the manufacturing process; Jennifer Michaux, senior development scientist; and Janera Harris, quality assurance manager—and he led us to the conference room for lunch. Ross and I handed out some pictures of Thomas and told the story of his short, precious life, and then Mark gave us a full presentation, complete with slides and photographs, on Cytonet's groundbreaking work.

Many biotech firms like to focus on treatments for common ailments, thereby maximizing their potential for profit. But Cytonet's work began with a much smaller focus—children under the age of five with a liver disease called a urea cycle disorder. Just one hundred children are born in the United States each year with this rare genetic disorder. The mutation causes a deficiency in one of the six liver enzymes whose job it is to remove nitrogen from the bloodstream and convert it to urea, which is transferred to the urine and safely exits the body. In urea cycle disorders, the nitrogen builds up as highly toxic ammonia, a life-threatening condition. If the ammonia in the blood reaches the brain, it can result in brain damage, coma, or even death. Most babies who receive this diagnosis die within a few weeks of birth.

There is no cure for this condition; a liver transplant is the only option. The catch is that newborns are too small to receive a transplant safely.

Therefore, instead of transplanting entire organs, the company has developed a method for isolating healthy liver cells and transplanting those into diseased organs; the transplanted cells will engraft into the recipient's liver and take up the work that the diseased liver cannot do.

Cytonet receives donated healthy livers that are unsuitable for transplantation—they may have been damaged in surgery or not completely flushed of blood, which causes bruising. The researchers have developed, and are constantly refining, a process by which they can extract cells from these healthy but nontransplantable organs. The first stage of the process introduces an enzyme called collagenase, which cleaves the collagen that holds the liver cells. What's left is a liquid form of the liver, which is then put into sterile bags.

There are a number of different cell types in the liver, and the ones they want to isolate for transplant are called hepatocytes. To get the hepatocytes, the bags are put into a simple centrifuge, which causes the heavier hepatocytes to fall to the bottom; the other cells float to the top and are then aspirated off.

The remaining hepatocytes are cryopreserved—a.k.a. frozen—until they can be injected into a recipient.

Cytonet is offered hundreds of livers every month from the fifty-eight OPOs across the country, but after weeding out organs that are very fatty or cirrhotic (the enzyme can't penetrate that kind of tissue), they are able to accept and use on average around just eight each month. Of those, approximately half go to what is called the manufacturing lab—where the livers are processed into sterile bags of hepatocytes ready for cell transplantation—and the other half go to the R & D lab, where they help refine and improve their processes. I didn't know which lab Thomas's liver went to, but I was grateful that it had made it through the Cytonet gauntlet of criteria. Being a Cytonet donor struck me as an elite status that many of us, probably me included, might never attain.

Cytonet's first milestone was the successful implementation of its liver-cell therapy in 2004. The recipient was a sixty-four-year-old woman who had eaten poisonous death cap mushrooms, the culprit in most human deaths by mushroom. The deadly fungus causes organ failure within days, but two weeks after she received liver-cell therapy the lucky woman went home.

The first four children with urea cycle disorders were treated in what are called therapeutic attempts, before the company had approval to begin a clinical trial. The patients—one in Italy and three in Germany—had no alternative treatment, so their physicians contacted Cytonet and asked the company to provide the liver cells; after receiving the cells, the physicians injected them into their patients. The company was able to use the anecdotal data from those four patients in their application to conduct a clinical study in Europe, the United States, and Canada. Another sixteen patients were successfully treated in that study. The youngest patient treated with this therapy was just six hours old.

Cytonet has since treated two patients with different kinds of rare liver metabolic disorder: One kind is Crigler-Najjar syndrome, an inherited condition caused by a malfunctioning enzyme that can lead to jaundice as well as muscle, nerve, and brain damage. The other is hyperoxaluria, which can result in lethal damage to the kidneys.

Starting in 2016, Cytonet plans to begin a new study for treating acute liver failure resulting from an external toxicity, such as might result from alcohol poisoning or an acetamino-phen overdose. Mark Johnston told us that the therapy is not suitable for patients with viruses such as hepatitis or cancer, since those diseases will also infect the transplanted donor cells. But in an otherwise healthy liver that has been damaged by some external toxicity—as was the case with the woman who ate the wrong mushrooms—the liver cell treatment gives the liver time to heal itself.

When I asked Mark why the company was so enthusias-tically focused on treating a disease with so few patients—he considers it lucky if Cytonet can treat fifteen to twenty patients a year—he said, "Our strategy was to go after this particular condition to prove the concept would work and was safe. Then we'll broaden it to other liver diseases." In the long run, the company hopes to not only take people off the organ-transplant waiting list, but perhaps eliminate the need for liver transplants altogether.

While we were eating lunch, the "liver phone" rang. The entire Cytonet team was on alert, because they were expecting an organ that was traveling from California. It was on the way.

I was impressed by all the systems that were in place to monitor everything. There was an extraordinary amount of thought going into every detail. Janera Harris explained that she was responsible for making sure that even the vendors of the medical supplies that the scientists at Cytonet used, like gloves and tubes, had the right quality-control measures in place.

After lunch, we took a tour through the facility and saw where Thomas's liver would have been prepared for the cell isolation procedure. We were shown a laminar airflow hood, which prevents contaminants in the air from touching the liver, and which I thought looked like the sneeze guard over a salad bar.

Mark had promised that I would be able to see liver cells under a microscope, but they would not be Thomas's. Before we arrived, Jennifer Michaux had taken some liver cells out of cryopreservation and magnified them for us to see on a computer monitor. For the Cytonet staff, looking at liver cells seemed like no big deal. But I had never seen real liver cells in my life, and I probably never would again. For me, this was a really special occasion.

As we walked through the staff break room to another part of the building, I was delighted to see that our visit had already had an impact on these busy people's lives: One of the pictures we had just distributed had been hastily taped to a whiteboard, with an arrow pointing to Thomas and these words handwritten in dry-erase marker:

Thomas Gray was a Cytonet donor. Died 3/29/10.

It had been so difficult for me to give away Thomas's organs and not know what happened to them. I imagined that it must be hard for researchers to receive an organ from a fellow human being and not feel some kind of curiosity, or sympathy, or connection. I took that message on the break room wall as a sign: they have been wondering about us, too.

During our lunch, we had learned that it was Sonya who received the package with Thomas's liver and, in fact, held my son's liver in her hands. Part of Sonya's job was validation, which means coming up with new ways to clean and freeze the liver cells, then testing these methods over and over and over to make sure they are really working.

Before we left, Mark looked up the liver-processing records from the week Thomas died. Though the name was not revealed, Mark found the records of a baby boy who had died on March 29, 2010, and whose liver was recovered and donated through WRTC. Since this was the only neonatal liver to arrive at Cytonet around that time, it was clear to me that the liver in this record was Thomas's.

When Thomas's liver arrived at Cytonet, it showed some signs of bruising, which was a result of pooled blood that could not be flushed out after surgery. Sometimes this is the result of an abnormality in the anatomy of the liver. As a result, his liver was not in the best condition for the cell isolation procedure for patient treatment purposes, so the cells were not injected into a baby with a urea cycle disorder. Instead, Thomas's liver was used in a study that Cytonet was performing on the ideal temperature for freezing neonatal liver cells. This study required the donation of six neonatal livers; that might not sound like much, but it took approximately five months for Cytonet to get all six. The child who had died on March 29, 2010, had donated liver number three.

I pictured Thomas as a member of a six-baby NBA dream team.

When the study was complete, it showed that neonatal liver cells can be frozen at the same temperature as adult and pediatric liver cells, which is minus 150 degrees Celsius. For the scientists, this information was vital for the work they were doing. From then on, minus 150 degrees Celsius would be a secretly special number to me.

"You remember that there are names, there are sisters and mothers and fathers of these donors," Sonya said that day. "It's not just a liver. Without the family making that sacrifice even though they know it's not going to another person directly—we have to remember that their sacrifice is helping someone else."

Though it was clear that the liver that arrived that day was Thomas's, we could never be 100 percent sure because of the agreement of confidentiality. We heard another story that brought home the challenges the staff faced in working with anonymous, or "de-identified," samples. One day, an employee was leafing through a copy of the Southwest Airlines in-flight magazine during a trip and stumbled across an ad for the Yale Medical School, touting its successful treatment of a baby with a new liver-cell therapy. Was this the Cytonet therapy? Though the scientists at Cytonet developed the process, they didn't interact directly with patients. The Cytonet staff could finally see the face of someone who just might be a patient.

Subsequently the *Yale Pediatric Update* published a story about the "first pediatric liver-cell transplantation in the Northeast." Dr. Sukru Emre, M.D., director of the Yale–New Haven Transplantation Center, performed the procedure on three-week-old Abbas Syed in 2010. Accompanying the article was a picture of Veena Chowdhan holding her laughing toddler.

Later, I would ask Dr. Emre about Abbas, and he would confirm that Abbas had been treated with donated hepatocytes from Cytonet. Abbas received hepatic cell infusions every day for six days. All the cells he received came from the liver of one unidentified deceased donor. This donation played a vital role in saving Abbas's life. This was especially poignant given that Veena and her husband had previously lost a baby girl to the same condition. When she learned that there was a new treatment that had worked for at least one patient in Germany, she jumped at the chance. Nine months after Abbas received the liver-cell therapy, he received, in an eleven-hour operation, his full liver transplant. As of early 2016, Abbas was a thriving and healthy kindergartener.

Although Thomas would not have been directly involved in this treatment, I couldn't help but feel a connection to Abbas and his family from that moment on.

At the end of our afternoon at Cytonet, we reluctantly removed our visitor badges and got back in the car to begin the long drive home. I felt physically exhausted, but emotionally buoyed by the new answers, new friends, and further evidence of human compassion. In school, science had been one of my worst subjects. I thought it was too difficult to understand and boring, but I was starting to see things differently. No, science was definitely not boring. To paraphrase Neil deGrasse Tyson, I started appreciating science as being something close to magic, except it's better: it's real.

Cytonet was the only for-profit research organization to receive one of Thomas's donations, and I wondered how I would feel about that. This visit helped me make up my mind. First and foremost, Cytonet is the only organization that wanted Thomas's liver. If Cytonet didn't want it, it would have been buried in the ground. So my choice had not been between donating to a for-profit and a nonprofit company. It was between a for-profit and nothing. From that perspective, we made the right choice for us: a donation to a for-profit company was better than a liver in the ground.

Also, Cytonet is directly saving lives. And as a parent, I know what it feels like to be desperate for any kind of help. When your child is sick, it doesn't matter if a company is nonprofit or for-profit. All that matters is the answer to the question, Can you save my child? For many children, Cytonet hepatocytes are a life-saving treatment, and their only option. Each liver donated to Cytonet produces a variable number of cells. In some cases, one liver will make enough cell infusions for one patient. In others, one liver can help multiple patients. At the time of this writing, one donor has the potential to save up to six lives.

Dietmar Hopp started investing in Cytonet and other bio-tech companies because he saw a void in government funding that he could fill himself. This privately funded company might be making breakthroughs faster than a nonprofit organization could. They were also the only ones taking on the financial risk if the project failed.

I wondered how I might feel about Thomas's donations going to a for-profit company. As I learned more about it, I came to understand that nonprofits and for-profits both have their strengths and weaknesses, and I feel proud to be connected to *all* the places that received Thomas's donations.

At this point, the journey was over. I had broken through the taboos and the confidentiality and met the actual research-ers who received Thomas's donations. In most cases I was the first donor family they had ever met.

People have asked me if I saw anything shady, or learned anything I wish I had not. I saw the opposite. I saw normal, hardworking, legitimate researchers going to work and doing research. It really is like it is on TV: the labs, the coats, the microscopes, the nerd jokes.

One of the biggest surprises to me was how immensely

admirable all of these projects are. These people are trying to cure cancer and other diseases. They don't act like it's a big deal, because they do it all day for years on end. But as an outsider, I was really impressed and honored to meet them and breathe the same air they did.

Thomas was their colleague. And now they could put a name to him. This meant everything.

CHAPTER TEN

Out of My Comfort Zone
Spring 2013

I had found great peace in completing my search for Thomas's donations. I knew he was contributing to the greater good. And Callum, now a toddler coming up on his third birthday, was thriving and a delight to have around. Everything was good. Ross and I started talking about having another baby.

But I was still processing everything that had happened. In the fall of 2012, I tried something new: I signed up for a storytelling class through an organization called Speakeasy DC. The class met one night a week, during which each of the ten students wrote and rehearsed telling a seven-minute story.

I decided to tell the story of touring Schepens. The final exam consisted of getting up onstage at a bar to tell our stories in public. I emailed invitations to the doctors and nurses at Inova Fairfax, where I'd had the babies, as well as everyone I'd met at Schepens. (I knew it was a long shot asking people from Boston to travel to DC, but they were the subjects of the story, and you never know.) In the end, Ross, Callum, my brothers Ethan and Mark—who recorded my performance on video—

and my friend Aimee came. It went pretty well, and I was proud of myself for being able to do it. Mark got a good recording, which I shared with the folks at WRTC so they could at least share my story with the team who worked so hard to make this donation happen.

So when I got a call in October 2012 from a journalist named Emily Berman from our local NPR station, WAMU, asking to interview me for a story about coping with the loss of a newborn, I was open to it. She had been referred to me by Kelly Gallo, the perinatal-concerns nurse who had worked with us. I had invited Kelly to the bar event. She hadn't been able to make it, but when Emily Berman asked her if she knew of any families who might be willing to speak with her for her story, Kelly gave her my name. On WAMU that day I told the story of the boys' birth and Thomas's anencephaly, as well as that first visit to meet Dr. Zieske and see Thomas at work at Schepens.

Then WRTC asked me to speak at a Donor Family Council meeting in December, and I jumped at the chance to tell other families how healing it had been to learn about my son's donation journey and meet all the people who were part of his life now.

In January I began the second-to-last course for my master's degree. This particular course was designed to coach students through the thesis project, and during the first week of class the professor handed out a worksheet and asked us to fill in information about our current job and career goals, with the idea that this exercise would help us focus on an appropriate thesis subject.

I was happy with my job at NISH, where I had started the AbilityOne Speakers Bureau. I had secured speaking opportunities for people who suffered from severe disabilities, whether they were born with them or acquired them as a result of disease or traumatic injury. The most popular speakers were veterans of the wars in Iraq and Afghanistan, and we also worked with people with Down syndrome, learning disabilities, mental illness, or other serious challenges. For all of them, I helped craft narratives about their lives, what it was like to find employment, and how much it mattered to them and their families that they were able to live independently. The job was never boring, and I liked helping these amazing people. After ten years, I was good at my job, and I had no plans to leave, so that's what I wrote under "current job."

But I also had to write something about my career goals, so, merely for something to say, I wrote: "Communications for an organ donation organization," since so much of my life in recent months had been taken up with the subject.

My answer brought to mind an article I had read some months earlier in the *New York Times* about a nondirected kidney-donation chain that had saved the lives of thirty people. A nondirected donor is also called a "Good Samaritan"—a person who donates a kidney anonymously to a stranger, in the same way that you might donate blood to a stranger. This donation can trigger some kidney-paired donations, which occur when living donor A wants to donate to loved one B but their blood types are incompatible, and living donor C wants to donate to recipient D, but their blood types don't match, either. The pairs essentially swap kidneys, with donor A giving to recipient D, and donor C giving to recipient B. The more I thought about it, the more I loved the topic, so it was perfect for my thesis. And it would be a privilege to interview these people personally.

Thanks to my personal experience with donation, I knew exactly how to start: I called Lisa Colaianni at WRTC and asked if she could help connect me with some living donors. Lisa herself had donated a kidney to a stranger, so she became my first interview subject. She then introduced me to seven more people, and they in turn introduced me to three more. Over the next three months, I interviewed ten people who had donated a kidney to a stranger. Many of them were involved in kidney chains, which means they helped to save the life of more than one person. One person I interviewed personally triggered a kidney chain that saved the lives of thirteen people.

As I completed my thesis research, I noticed a phenomenon: some of the donors reported feeling helpless because of the death of a loved one at some point before their kidney donation. There was nothing they could do to stop the illness and death of their family member or dear friend, but there was something they could do to save the life of a stranger. Donating a kidney to a stranger helped them even the odds with the universe and feel powerful again. I nicknamed it "retribution donation." It was like saying to the universe, "You took my loved one for no reason, so I'm going to save this other person for no reason."

It was an honor to talk to these donors. Thomas's death had made me understand how cruel life can be, and nondirected kidney donation is an example of how wonderful life can be.

During the semester, WRTC approached me a few more times to do more speaking engagements for them, including at a board of directors meeting. After one speech to the WRTC staff, a clinical-recovery coordinator, Elizabeth Turner, introduced herself; she had been in the room when Thomas's eyes were removed. It was emotional and delightful to meet her. I met other parents of donors, and saw how donation helped them cope with their loss. Although they didn't have the choice to save their loved ones, they felt empowered that they at least had the choice and power to help someone else—literally saving the lives of strangers. And I had seen the healing power of meeting the unknown recipients. I heard that some recipients didn't want to meet their donor's family, and I was puzzled. What were they scared of?

I found myself requesting personal time off from my job at NISH to do these events at WRTC. I started to think, *If I'm taking time off from my job to work another job instead of relaxing or going on a vacation, maybe it's a sign that I should get that other job.*

As if by magic, a job opened up as a director of marketing and public affairs at the American Association of Tissue Banks. During a phone interview with Frank Wilton, the president and CEO of AATB, I found that I was excited just to be able to talk about the subject, and the more we talked, the more I realized it was perfect: I was already doing media and advocacy, and I knew all about donation.

And that's how I got my dream job before I'd even finished the course that had asked me to identify my dream job.

I was thirty-nine years old, and I'd thought I would stay in my old job forever, but here I was in a new job at AATB, and with a lot to learn.

For a start I had to familiarize myself with the world of tissue banking, which is complex. When Frank recommended I read a large spiral-bound book called *The Standards of Tissue Banking,* I thought to myself, *I was going to read it anyway.* Everything he gave me to read intrigued me; the job made me feel newly alive.

Medical advancements are constantly changing, as I learned those first few months trying to get up to speed.

There are more than a million tissue transplants in the United States every year, and many of them transform the patient's life. Patients who were not able to walk or work are able to maintain their independence once again after receiving a transplant of just a few millimeters of ligament, or a bone chip, from a stranger.

Upon death, one person can donate up to eight organs: heart, lungs, kidneys, liver, pancreas, intestines; and, if you add in tissue—bones, corneas, skin, tendons, ligaments, cartilage, valves, nerves, veins—hundreds more recipients can benefit.

A donated heart valve can replace an adult's damaged valve or correct a baby's congenital defect.

A bone graft from a donor's femur can be reconfigured into a vertebra to correct a spinal deformity.

Bones, tendons, and ligaments lost or damaged by cancer, trauma, degenerative joint disease, or arthritis can all be replaced.

Burn survivors need donated skin, which is used as a dressing to prevent infection while their own skin heals.

Professional athletes who get ulnar collateral ligament (UCL) reconstruction, or Tommy John surgery, are sometimes the recipients of donor tissue, often referred to as an "allograft."

But tissue banking is not only about the donations of someone who has died. Living donors can donate reproductive tissue such as sperm and oocytes (eggs). Mothers who have delivered a baby can donate the afterbirth, which includes the umbilical cord, placenta, and amnion. This is referred to as "birth tissue," and it can be processed into skin grafts for burn survivors. At the time of this writing, depending on the size, one placenta can be processed into healing skin grafts for up to four different people.

One thing I noticed—and didn't like at all—was how often the term *cadaver* is used instead of *donor*. I never, ever, think of my son as a "cadaver," and I cringe at the thought that someone else might. I learned that I am not the only donor mom to be offended by this usage. The National Kidney Foundation's Donor Family Council started the effort to eliminate the words *harvest* and *cadaver* from the transplant lexicon in the 1990s. Major newspapers and medical journals, such as the *American Journal of Transplantation,* have since adopted less offensive language, too. One of the first things I worked on at AATB was a document for the media called "Communicating with Care and Respect." The AATB is one of many organizations that encourage the use of the term *deceased donor* as opposed to *cadaver.*

A part of my job would entail working with Donate Life America, a nonprofit alliance of organizations around the country dedicated to promoting organ, eye, and tissue donation. Donate Life America essentially serves as the marketing arm of the United Network for Organ Sharing, or UNOS. UNOS, which is referred to as "the computer in the sky," contains the algorithm that assigns available organs—and now vascularized composite grafts (including limbs and, now, faces)—to patients who need one.

Before UNOS was founded, individual hospitals and local organ-procurement organizations handled organ recoveries and transplants. But if an organ could not be used locally, there was no way to find a recipient elsewhere in a timely manner, and much-needed organs went unused while patients in need languished or died. In 1977, the first computerized database was started, and as more and more hospitals started doing transplants, Congress passed the National Organ Transplant Act in 1984 to create a national network, and thus UNOS was born.

In 1992, UNOS was instrumental in setting up the Coalition on Donation, now known as Donate Life America, as an independent nonprofit to encourage donor registration. Nearly thirty thousand organ transplants were done in 2014, but more than 100,000 people needed one. There are currently more than 120,000 people on the waiting list for an organ transplant in the United States, including more than 2,000 children. Every ten minutes another name is added to the list, and more than twenty people die every day waiting.

A couple of months after I started work at AATB, the CEO, Frank Wilton, thought it would be a good idea to introduce me to the people at Donate Life America in person, so we planned a trip to Richmond, Virginia, where DLA is based, a few blocks from the UNOS offices, where we would also pay a visit.

Before we left, I said to Frank, "This isn't officially related to AATB business, but could we swing by Old Dominion Eye Foundation? That's where my son's eyes went." Frank agreed, and I set up a meeting with Christina Jenkins, the associate director and director of public relations.

Helen Keller herself inspired the formation of Old Dominion Eye Foundation when she spoke at a Lions Club event and founder Melvin Jones was in the audience.

Melvin Jones was a businessman living in Chicago who had been elected to a leadership position with the Business Circle, a group of businessmen who had lunch together and helped advance one another's financial interests. Jones felt that these meetings were a misuse of influence, talent, and ambition, so he used his leadership position to change the direction of the group, inviting the members to help improve their communities instead. Jones famously said, "You can't get very far until you start doing something for somebody else." In 1917, tired of the Business Circle's meager aims, Melvin Jones helped establish the Lions Club, the charitable organization that now has chapters around the world and nearly half a million members.

By the mid-1920s, activist, speaker, and author—as well as suffragette and unapologetic Socialist—Helen Keller had already both established the Helen Keller International organization and helped found the ACLU. Keller had gone blind and deaf at age nineteen months after a severe illness. The first deaf and blind person to get a degree, she toured extensively, advocating for people with disabilities. One of her stops was at the 1925 International Convention of Lions Clubs in Cedar Point, Ohio, where she asked the Lions Clubs to focus their efforts and take on the cause of helping people who are blind.

"I appeal to you, Lions," she said, "you who have your sight, your hearing, you who are strong and brave and kind. Will you not constitute yourselves Knights of the Blind in this crusade against darkness?"

And so they did. The support of efforts to help people see has been a central tenet of the Lions Clubs ever since. And the Old Dominion Eye Foundation, Inc., was founded in 1962 with the help of the Lions Clubs.

It was a long way from Melvin Jones and Helen Keller, but as with so much of what happened with Thomas, I realized that his donation was part of a long line of such acts—acts of service that could move forward only when like-minded people got together and decided to "start doing something for somebody else." More than thirty-three thousand donations have been processed by Old Dominion since those early days, and more than fifteen thousand people have had their sight restored through transplant, thanks to all of the people who helped establish the ODEF.

I learned that Thomas's eyes were recovered by 7:30 A.M. on Monday, March 29, at Children's National Medical Center, by David Taylor, the branch manager for the Old Dominion Eye Foundation at their Fairfax, Virginia, office. The corneas were then transported to the ODEF's Richmond, Virginia, headquarters and arrived the next day: Tuesday, March 30. In Richmond, they were checked, cleared for defects and scars, and prepared for shipping by Jennifer Payton, the lab coordinator. Her signature appears on Thomas's paperwork. That afternoon, the corneas left ODEF for Schepens Eye Research Institute in Boston via Federal Express. They arrived in Boston on Wednesday, March 31—the day of Thomas's funeral.

On a sunny August day Frank and I arrived at the brick building on Arboretum Drive that houses ODEF. We were greeted by the hugely smiling faces of Christina Jenkins and ODEF's executive director, Bill Proctor. They exuded welcome and excitement. Bill has been in the profession for thirty-five years and is a leader in the field. Early in his career, he worked closely with the National Eye Institute in Washington, D.C., and he saw firsthand the impact of research and the need for research tissue.

I believe it's because of Bill Proctor's passion for research that Thomas was able to donate. It turns out we were very lucky that we lived in Washington so that we were in range of ODEF. Had we lived in a different part of the country, or had Thomas died elsewhere, his eyes likely would not have been recovered, because infant corneas aren't suitable for transplant. They are too flimsy, and many eye banks will not recover tissue that is not suitable for transplant, even though such tissue is extremely valuable for research and there is often a waiting list for it.

Like many eye banks around the country, ODEF has a mission statement that includes donation for transplant as well as research. But since a single cornea intended for transplant is reimbursed approximately three thousand dollars, and a cornea for research is reimbursed only a tenth of that, tissue for transplant is the main goal of most eye banks. When eye tissue is not suitable for transplant, sometimes organ-procurement organizations forget to even ask about research opportunities. And many eye banks and OPOs have a practice of recovering for research only if a family specifically asks.

But research tissue is no second-class citizen at ODEF.

Thanks to some funding ODEF receives from the Lions Clubs, ODEF can afford to procure eye tissue for research without as much concern for the reimbursement of processing fees. (Although most eye banks are nonprofit, they still need to cover the expenses of equipment, accreditation fees, training, and staff.)

ODEF works closely with WRTC, which covers Washington, DC, and northern Virginia, as well as LifeNet Health, which is the OPO for southern Virginia. When either group gets a call from a hospital that a potential donor has died or is likely to soon, they reach out to ODEF. ODEF then checks its own database first to see what corneal transplants are waiting, and then its database of local research projects. They also work closely with the National Disease Research Interchange (NDRI), since they keep a national registry of research projects.

At Old Dominion I presented pictures of Thomas and the researchers we met, and afterward Bill Proctor said, "I've always known that research was vital, but meeting you, hearing your experience, really brings it home. Thank you."

During our tour, Bill showed us the microscope they use to do visual inspections of the corneas. Corneas are checked for signs of damage, disease, and scarring. In 2013, corneas with a LASIK scar were less likely to be used for transplant, so ODEF donated them to doctors in other countries, such as Egypt. Today, there are two new processes—Descemet's stripping endothelial keratoplasty (DSEK), and Descemet's membrane endothelial keratoplasty (DMEK)—that allow some LASIK-scarred corneas to be transplanted. Instead of removing and replacing the entire cornea, which can contain a LASIK scar, a smaller part of the cornea that does not include the scar is recovered and used for transplant.

Bill also explained that humans are born with perhaps six

thousand or seven thousands cells in their corneas, and that number diminishes with age. ODEF has a general guideline that acceptable corneas for transplant should have a minimum of two thousand cells. Corneas with lower counts are more likely to be shipped overseas or sent for research, and the initial count is done right here at ODEF.

And then I was introduced to Jennifer Payton, who had become a mythical figure in my son's life.

I was overwhelmed with emotion when I met Jennifer, because she had processed Thomas's eyes.

As ever, I was the first donor mom she'd ever met. As soon as we could, Jennifer and I quietly sneaked away from the group. I wanted to know how eyes were recovered (that was part of her job, too), so she took me to her lab, where she showed me a package the size of a manicure kit with the recovery tools inside. It was simpler, and even more fascinating, than I'd imagined.

After the tour, we all went to Carytown, a trendy neighborhood in Richmond, and had lunch at a French bistro. The ODEF staff said that most of them had never met a donor's family before—a refrain I was getting so used to hearing. As we talked, I realized that it was these people, sitting at this table, who had made Thomas's donation possible, and my heart swelled with gratitude.

"We're going to go back to work refreshed to keep doing what we do," said Christina. "I think we needed this."

You and me both, I thought.

I stayed in touch with the staff at ODEF; Bill invited me to speak at their 2014 annual meeting. He told me later that a number of the board members remarked that they hadn't fully believed him all the years he'd been advocating for the importance of donating for research until they heard Thomas's story.

These meetings seemed like one of those rare cases of a true win-win.

Back at home, Ross was supportive of my new line of work, and he was glad to learn about the difference that Thomas was still making. As parents, we got a lot of questions about when we would tell Callum about his brother. We decided early on that we would never lie about Thomas's existence, or hide the facts from Callum. To me, being an identical twin is part of Callum's identity, and it would have felt strange to keep it from him. Also, baby photographs from the hospital revealed two children; there was no hiding that there was another baby in the bassinet with him. But why *would* we hide it? Thomas's death was simply something that happened, not something to be ashamed of or embarrassed about. We decided to display two photos of Thomas in our home, and we made a book of photographs of Callum and Thomas together to share with Callum.

Ross and I continued to visit Thomas's grave a few times a year—on his birthday, or if we happened to be driving that way. When Callum first started learning to talk, he asked us some fascinating and heartbreaking questions: "Is Thomas scared under the stone?" "Will he ever come out and play with me?" We answer the questions as honestly as we can. We told him Thomas will never come play because he died. Everyone in the world will die at some point. A lot of people are older when they die, but people can die anytime, even when they are young. Sometimes young kids get sick or have an accident and that is just part of life. None of us knows when we will die, but it's okay to die. Maybe we will even see Thomas when we die.

One day I was talking to little Callum, and I told him that some people say there is a place called Heaven.

"What is it like in Heaven?" Callum asked.

"I don't know. No one has been there and come back," I

told him. "Nobody knows for sure. What do you think happens there?"

"Look it up on your phone," he said.

At a loss, I bought a book called *What Is Heaven,* by Maria Shriver, and read it to him. A few months later, after a trip to Scotland, he came back to the subject.

"Mommy, remember that book that said Heaven is above the clouds?"

"Yes."

"Well, that's not true. Because I was on an airplane, and I was above the clouds, and I did not see any people."

On the twins' third birthday, we planned to stop by Thomas's grave and leave flowers. I told Callum he could draw a picture or write a note for his brother that we could leave on the grave. He drew one portrait of him and his brother eating french fries at McDonald's, and another of the two of them under a tent, camping.

That day, I asked him what he had wished for when he blew out his birthday candles, and he said, "I wish Thomas would be able to walk and play with me." It touched my heart and broke it at the same time. He saw other people who had a brother, and he wanted one, too. Things were beginning to sink in; he was starting to understand something about life, and about death.

What do you say to a child who wants to play with someone who is dead? All I could think of to say was, "Are you sure you don't you want Legos or something else?"

One day, Callum asked me if Thomas was still his brother even though he was dead, and I said yes. These moments were poignant, but not impossible to face. Perhaps in the past it was more common for young children to have a personal experience coping with death. In some countries, that is still a common experience. In modern-day America, it seems unusual. The topic is taboo, and we choose not to discuss it; but this can be isolating to a person who is grieving. I wanted to show Callum that coping with death is a normal part of life, and that feeling sad is normal.

By the time he was four, Callum had been to four family funerals: Thomas's; that of my stepfather, Bob; and those of both of my maternal grandparents. As he processed these events, he went through an interesting phase. For a few months, Callum would lie flat on the floor and say, "Pretend I'm under a stone. Put flowers on me." Whereas this might be cause for alarm in another family, it made sense in ours. This is a child who regularly visited a grave, in a safe environment with his family. The same way he playacted other events from his real life—like pretending to give us flu shots, or dental cleanings, or haircuts—he was also asking us to playact a funeral. Why not? I pretended to put flowers on him.

"Cry!" he giggled, pleased with his new game. "Be sad!"

"Waaaah!" I fake-cried. "I miss Callum so much."

"Now you go under a stone. Your turn."

Once, Callum said to me, "You have one son in Heaven and one son on earth."

"I guess that's true, yes."

"Do you know who else is in Heaven? Cheez-it."

I repeated the word quietly to myself a few times before I got it. He wasn't talking about crackers; he was talking about Jesus.

As a result of our open discussions, Callum is pretty matter-of-fact about his missing brother. We were having a family portrait taken one summer during a seaside vacation, and the photographer asked Callum, "Do you have any pets?"

"No, but I have a brother who died."

While Callum seems okay with it, grown-ups are occasionally taken aback by the open way he talks about Thomas. It reminds me of the way a generation or two ago people would say the word *cancer* in a whisper, as though it were scandalous.

Even though Thomas isn't here, Callum enlists him when he's feeling a bit mischievous. He'll run up behind me and slap me, and I'll turn around and say, "Who was that?"

"That was Thomas."

And like all brothers, Callum is protective of Thomas. If someone asks me how many children I have and Callum hears me answer, "One," he'll jump in and say, "No, no, you have two. You forgot about Thomas!"

I hope when Callum is older he'll fully understand that, no, I haven't forgotten about Thomas.

I'll never forget about him.

AMALYA'S STORY

Mortui vivos docent

Bethany Conkel was eleven weeks pregnant when she and her husband, Eric, received the devastating news that their child had anencephaly—the same neural tube defect that Thomas had. The Conkels, who are committed Christians, decided to carry the pregnancy to term and make the most they could out of their child's life and death.

"We felt from the very beginning of the pregnancy, even before we received the diagnosis, that the Lord was going to do something very special with this baby," Bethany said.

At fifteen weeks, they learned they were expecting a boy. The first step, then, was to pick a name with significance: they chose Amalya, a Hebrew word that means "work of the Lord," and for his middle name they chose Nathaniel, which means "given by God."

The Conkels thought about the kinds of things they would like to do with their son and drew up a bucket list: go to a local park with a long slide, go to a baseball game with Grandpa Dan, go camping, kayaking, to the zoo, to a monster-truck show—and, most especially, go on a visit to a Waffle House, where Bethany and Eric went after their wedding and where they continued to celebrate anniversaries. They decided to do these things "with Amalya" while he was in utero.

At the time of the diagnosis, Eric was an undergraduate studying physical therapy and working in the anatomy lab at the University of Dayton, in Dayton, Ohio. He had seen firsthand how much the students learned from one donated human body, and his experience as a student gave the Conkels the idea to donate.

Bethany and Eric called universities near their Dayton home, including the University of Dayton, Wright State University, and the University of Cincinnati. They were stunned to learn that there was no need for a neonatal donor. In one instance, Bethany was told that studying an infant would be too emotionally difficult for the medical students.

Bethany and Eric then called hospitals, thinking there would be a need for Amalya's body for practice surgery or research. Again, the answer was no.

Bethany asked the genetic specialist who had given her Amalya's diagnosis if she knew of any options for donation. She didn't, but she provided Bethany with the contact information for Life Connections of Ohio, the federally designated nonprofit organ-procurement organization for northwestern and West Central Ohio.

Bethany called Life Connections and learned there might be a possibility for a tissue donation—Amalya's heart valves—if he met certain weight requirements at birth. However, regular ultrasounds during the course of the pregnancy showed that Amalya would likely be too small.

Bethany wondered whether there was anything else she could do. She wasn't going to give up until she knew for sure.

Life Connections offered to contact their partner, the International Institute for the Advancement of Medicine, or IIAM, to inquire about research donation options for the Conkels. IIAM was founded in 1986 and partners with fifty-five organ-procurement organizations across the country to connect available specimens with the researchers who need them.

But weeks passed, and Bethany heard nothing.

Bethany's C-section was scheduled for September 10, and on

September 5 she called Life Connections of Ohio one last time, just to see if they had any news for her.

"I'm so sorry; things are not working out," her contact explained. "Every door is shut. There are no suitable research placements. Your baby is too small to donate for transplant. We're really sorry."

That evening, she told Eric, "I'm at peace. I know we've done everything possible. Let's just enjoy the last few days with our baby."

But after a few restless nights, Bethany realized that she really wasn't at peace. On September 7, Bethany called the 800 number on IIAM's website and reached the call-center answering service. She asked about whole-body donations, and explained the urgency.

"Let me find someone who can help you," said the call-center representative.

A few hours later, Bethany finally got the call she and Eric had been waiting for. The IIAM rep told her that they had found research placements for Amalya's liver, pancreas, and whole body. In order to donate, Bethany would be required to sign a consent form, complete a medical and social history interview to disclose events in Bethany's life that may have exposed the baby to infectious disease, and provide a sample of blood on-site at Life Connections of Ohio—only five miles from their house. Heavily pregnant but delighted, Bethany asked her father if he would drive her there.

Bethany happily completed the paperwork and answered some personal questions—such as "How many sexual partners have you had?"—in front of her father.

"Fortunately, I have a pretty open relationship with my dad, so it was nothing he didn't already know," she laughed. By the time she got home, she felt relief washing over her.

"We were able to enjoy that last weekend with our son, knowing that we'd done everything to make the most of his short life. Now we were going to be able to make the most of his death as well."

On September 10, 2012, Amalya Nathaniel Conkel was born by C-section at Miami Valley Hospital in Dayton, Ohio, at 7:51 A.M.

As soon as he was born, the doctor laid him on Bethany's chest.

"He's so precious," she said to Eric. "I wasn't expecting him to be this precious."

Eric helped clean his body and place him on the scale. He was four pounds, nine ounces. As the doctor sutured her incision, Bethany and Eric told Amalya how much they loved him and how special he was. Both Bethany and Eric held Amalya to their chests for skin-to-skin contact. Once the surgery was complete, the new family of three joined the extended family in a private hospital room. Amalya's eyes were open, but he did not move or cry. Six grandparents and three great-grandparents were able to hold him while he was still alive, and a total of nine aunts and uncles were able to meet him.

After an hour, Bethany felt a mother's intuition. Though there were no outward signs, Bethany felt it in her heart.

"Oh, Eric," Bethany said. "He's leaving us."

The nurse checked Amalya's heartbeat; it was at only five beats per minute. Bethany's dad, a pastor, laid his hand on his grandson and said a prayer as Amalya passed away in Bethany's embrace at approximately 9:10 A.M.

"I know he felt our love," Bethany said. "His entire life was spent in the arms of those who cared for him deeply."

In the moments after he died, family members held him and said their good-byes. Then Eric carried his son down the hospital corridor to the operating room, where a special team of surgeons was waiting to recover Amalya's pancreas, his liver, and the blood from his heart. The surgery took about two hours. Once the recovery was complete, they sutured Amalya's flesh down the front of his sternum, covered it with a bandage, and dressed him.

A doctor returned Amalya's body to his family. The Conkels were told that the recovery went well and the organs were in great condition for the researchers.

"We were thrilled," said Bethany.

The Conkels were joined by twenty-seven friends and family members and spent the rest of the day taking pictures of Amalya, making prints of his hands and feet, and giving him lots of hugs and kisses.

"We even had a birthday party complete with cupcakes, a 'birthday boy' hat, a 'zero' candle, and a tear-filled round of 'Happy Birthday,'" said Bethany. "Joy overflowed from our room that day. I can't even describe in words what it was like."

Because the Conkels chose to participate in whole-body donation, Amalya's body needed to be cooled within twelve hours of his passing. Each family member said a final good-bye and then left Bethany and Eric to have a private moment with their son.

"Finally, we called for the nurse and handed our sweet boy over for the last time. The moment I let him go, my heart shattered. It was the hardest thing I've ever had to do. I was so in love with this sweet gift from the Lord, but I knew it was time for him to fulfill the rest of his purpose here on this earth."

Because of all the confidentiality protocols, all the Conkels knew was that Amalya would be studied by researchers somewhere in the United States. They wondered who would hold him next. That's when Bethany got an idea.

"Do you have a marker? A black Sharpie or something?" Bethany asked Eric. "I want to write a note to the researchers."

Eric searched his backpack.

"All I have are these two highlighters," Eric said, holding up one pink and one green one.

"They'll do," Bethany said.

Eric and Bethany each made a thumbprint in the shape of a

heart, and under each one wrote "Mom" and "Dad" in green. Below the hearts, they wrote in pink, "We hope he helps. Use him well."

Bethany and Eric left the maternity ward for home two days later. They were led through a back door so they didn't have to walk past the happy new families in the lobby.

On the way home, Bethany's phone rang. It was 11 A.M.

"We just wanted to let you to know that Amalya's flight has departed. He is on his way to the research facility now." Bethany Conkel felt a glimmer of hope.

Over the weeks that followed, Bethany and Eric learned more about where their son's donations went. Amalya's cord blood was sent to the Duke anencephaly study, where Thomas's and Callum's cord blood had gone. Blood from his heart and a small sample of his skin was sent to the Coriell Cell Repository in Camden, New Jersey, to develop cell lines to be stored for future research studies. His liver went to a university in the United States to study liver disease, including cirrhosis. His pancreas went to another university in the United States for the study of pediatric diabetes. And the rest of his body went to an emergency-medicine facility in Texas.

In many cases, a donated whole body is studied by medical students to learn about every structure of the human anatomy. A deceased donor whose body has had some of the organs removed is not suitable for this kind of study. However, Amalya's body, which was missing the liver and pancreas, was a suitable match for a special research project that involved the skeletal structure.

When an ER patient is dehydrated or in shock, his or her veins can collapse. When a vein can't be accessed, paramedics have another option: they can use a drill-like device to make a small hole in the patient's bone. This technique, called intraosseous access, or IO, was developed in 1922 by Dr. Henry Drinker, who first showed that it could work on, of all things, a rabbit. During World War II, the technique was used in the European theater to treat combat injuries.

Then, in 1984, James Orlowski, a physician from the renowned Cleveland Clinic who was working in India during a cholera outbreak, wrote an article in the *Archives of Pediatric and Adolescent Medicine* entitled "My Kingdom for an Intravenous Line." In it, Dr. Orlowski lamented, "There is nothing more exasperating than the inability to establish intravenous (IV) access in a critically ill child." Having repeatedly faced sick children with no "visible or palpable veins," Orlowski advocated for intraosseous access, since just about any medication or fluid such as saline or blood could be administered this way safely because a bone is essentially a large vein that will not collapse.

As a result of Orlowski's advocacy, IO was widely adopted in the United States for use in children, whose veins are smaller and can be more difficult to access through IV. For years, the most commonly accepted application site for pediatric cases was the tibia— the shin bone.

Scotty Bolleter, chief of the Office of Clinical Direction at the Centre for Emergency Health Science at Bulverde Spring Branch Emergency Medical Services in Spring Branch, Texas, is a passionate advocate of furthering the course of emergency medicine— and of improving the IO method. A veteran EMT and paramedic, he has trained thousands of physicians, nurses, physician assistants, and members of the military in what are called "advanced skills," although Bolleter considers them fundamental skills: the techniques for saving a soldier injured in combat or the next patient brought into the ER by ambulance. In partnership with a company called Vidacare, Scotty redesigned the IO technology in a device they named the EZ-IO. This is a handheld device, about the size and shape of a hot-glue gun, with a thin, 1.5-inch needle at the end.

According to Bolleter, the tibia was not the best location to establish IO, because the compartments in the muscles near the tibia are in close proximity to the bone, and if the needle is not placed perfectly into the bone, these compartments will swell. This buildup in pressure is called compartment syndrome, and it can lead to the death of a muscle and even the loss of a leg.

Bolleter proposed an alternative location: the femur. The muscles around the femur do not have the same properties as the those around the tibia and do not cause as much swelling if a needle is badly placed. As a result, the risk of compartment syndrome decreases—and evidence from tests indicated that the femur bone allowed better fluid flow in any case.

Bolleter would need to prove this to the FDA in a process called a Premarket Notification 510(k) clearance. This is the process by which the FDA determines whether the new device is similar to a device that has already been approved by the FDA, and therefore does not need an entirely new and lengthy clearance.

"The 510(k) process is like, 'Hey, Mom, that guy is doing it. Can I do it, too?'" said Scotty.

Bolleter and his Vidacare colleagues submitted their first 510(k) application for FDA approval of the femur location in 2007, and received their first rejection later that year, citing "lack of definitive proof" as the reason and asking for more detail. Bolleter was frustrated and heartbroken, but something kept him going.

"It had to be done," Scotty said. He tried to think of something—anything—that might prove to the FDA what he knew to be true. In 2002 or 2003, he had tested the EZ-IO on two different deceased children—a girl and a toddler boy. But because both children had been embalmed, the fluid flow did not offer a realistic example of how the flow would proceed in real life, so his tests had limited usefulness.

"The adult world rapidly embraced the use of the drill, but they were worried about the pediatric uses. 'It's too powerful—you will never be able to safely use this on a child,' and that kind of thing. They were scared," Scotty explained.

It occurred to Bolleter that in order to show how the EZ-IO would really work in the real world, he would need to demonstrate the device on an unembalmed pediatric human cadaver.

"Infant donors are hard to get. It's not that the researchers do not want these donors. It's the lack of access. They are not available," he said. Scotty placed a request for a deceased pediatric donor with the University of Texas Science Center in 2004.

Then he waited eight years.

In September 2012, Bolleter finally received a call asking if he would accept a neonatal donor from IIAM. By this time, not only was Bolleter still working on the EZ-IO, but he had an additional research project on airway management. He was trying to teach EMTs the differences between the airway of an adult and the airway of a child, and he figured that this donor might be able to help both studies.

Less than a week later, Amalya's body arrived via air freight at the Vidacare facility in Shavano, Texas. Bolleter and a member of his team opened the cardboard box labeled Human Remains. Inside was a casket covered with frozen gel packs. And inside the casket lay tiny Amalya.

"I wasn't shocked," Scotty said. "He looked peaceful, like he was resting. It was unusual that he had a note written on his clothing, but it was welcome. The way I run my division, we are open to families and the discussion.

"The folks who work in human anatomy—we talk to specimens. We know all their names; we use their names. If we are pulling someone out of a cooler and their head falls hard on the table—well, my staff apologizes immediately. It's not like slinging meat. We treated Amalya the same way we treat all of our specimens."

Scotty Bolleter considers himself lucky to have been taught this way. Throughout his training in health care, his teachers and professional mentors all treated deceased donors with care and reverence. He described a funeral at medical school where solemn physicians and nurse practitioners gathered to honor their "first patients" and say a silent "thank you" for what they would not have learned otherwise.

Scotty Bolleter had waited eight years for this donor, and he didn't know when he might get this chance again. Bolleter's team took as many pictures and videos as they could, including among their subjects the newly designed EZ-IO device as it was placed into Amalya's femur and as it released fluid. Using fluorography—photography using fluorescence—Bolleter was able to successfully record and display the flow of fluid into Amalya's bone using the EZ-IO. Even then, he wondered if these images might be the evidence the FDA needed to understand that this device had the potential to save human lives.

During the procedure, Amalya's airway was also closely studied. Securing an airway quickly can be a matter of life and death in emergency medicine, and the airway of a child, especially the epiglottis, is different from that of an adult or a training dummy. Bolleter took pictures of Amalya's epiglottis and trachea to show other medical professionals exactly what it looks like to place a chest tube into such a tiny airway. These images would be incorporated into teaching tools and presentations that would be shared with thousands of professionals and students all over the world.

In the meantime, Bethany contacted IIAM to see if there were any updates from the researchers.

She got some surprising news.

"Never in a million years did I think I would get this," Bethany said. Vidacare had provided a two-page handwritten note to IIAM to be delivered to Amalya's parents.

"Dear Mom & Dad," it opened. The letter expressed condolences for their loss and gratefulness for their generosity. It explained that Amalya already had a complete set of X-rays and was part of a research and education effort that involved intraosseous vascular access. His contribution would undoubtedly save the lives of some of the world's smallest and sickest patients. It closed with a plea that the parents never underestimate the magnitude of their son's gift. At the bottom were seven individual signatures from members of the team, and handwritten messages reading "God Bless You" and "God Bless You and Yours."

Bethany and Eric were floored. They read and reread the letter, and called her parents with the exciting news. The proud mom and dad created Christmas gifts for the researchers, which included a Christmas ornament and one of Amalya's handprints.

Nine months later, a rep from IIAM called the Conkels to let them know that the Vidacare research was done. Amalya's remains and his belongings would be returned to his family.

"Before the specimens go to be cremated, I write on their shroud the medical symbol for 'with'—a C with a line on top—and a heart, for love," said Scotty Bolleter.

In May 2013, the Conkels received a package at their Dayton home via Federal Express. Inside was a gold-colored box, about the size of a box that a bracelet might come in, affixed with a white label that read "This package contains the Cremated remains of Amalya Nathaniel Conkel." Inside the box was cotton batting and a sealed plastic bag filled with ashes. Also included in the package was Amalya's onesie with the message written in highlighter, his blanket, his hat, and some gifts from Vidacare: a cloth angel figurine, a knitted set of booties and a hat from an organization called Threads of Love, and a music CD.

Later that year, on October 30, 2013, Vidacare submitted the FDA approval application again, for the third time and with fingers crossed that these images would provide the evidence that was needed. Just over three months later, on February 11, 2014, the FDA published what is officially titled 510(k) NO: K132583 (TRADITIONAL). After seven years, three applications, and binders full of FDA questions and Vidacare responses, the FDA finally approved the use of the EZ-IO in the femur of children.

"The reviewer for the United States government specifically said, had it not been for those images, he likely would not have approved this particular usage," said Scotty Bolleter. Through word of mouth, Bolleter already knows for sure of one child whose life was saved by this device and this location.

For the Conkels, hearing about all this was a dream come true. Through their donation, they were able to spare another family the loss that they faced. Amalya's death had not been in vain.

But that is not all Amalya Nathaniel Conkel accomplished. The images and videos of Amalya's airway have appeared before thousands of medical professionals in educational presentations and publications in countries all over the world, from New Zealand to Syria. Scotty Bolleter said that in the year 2015 alone, he personally presented Amalya's images to at least ten thousand medical professionals, including the attendees of the Special Operations Medical Association's annual conference, a gathering of professionals from the fields of wilderness, austere, and disaster medicine.

Scotty Bolleter and the Conkels were able to meet face to face in August 2014, at the Musculoskeletal Transplant Foundation's leadership summit in New Orleans, and they presented him with one of Amalya's handprints.

"Only once have I ever met a family before the Conkels, and you get a chance to say how they made a difference," said Scotty. "Being able to complete that circle is critical; it allows you to move on the next important thing."

"It was amazing to be able to meet him in person, and very fulfilling," said Bethany.

For Bethany and Eric Conkel, donation brought healing. It gave Bethany what she called "Proud Mommy moments." "One of the hard parts about losing a baby at birth," Bethany said, "is that you don't get to watch them grow up; you don't get to watch them reach their first milestones, take their first steps, say their first words, eat their first food. But donation allowed us to be proud of our son in a different way."

On the third anniversary of receiving Amalya's diagnosis, Bethany did something special to honor her son. Moved by the FDA approval, Bethany got a tattoo. Just above her kneecap, where the newly approved insertion site is, she has a delicately drawn heart that comes to a point in an *A*—for Amalya.

And Bethany wasn't the only one recognizing Amalya.

"I have Amalya's handprint in my office, facing east," said Scotty Bolleter. "So the sun rises in his little handprint. He is representative of all of the donors that have come before and will come after. When I look at little Amalya's hand, I think of all the donors who work here. It's not just a carcass. It's not just a body laying on a table."

Scotty Bolleter is passionate about the contributions of these "voiceless teachers," and frustrated by the shortage of deceased donors that are available for crucial, life-saving research.

"Think about the images that da Vinci drew—*The Mechanics of Man*. Those people are dead, but the images look like they were drawn yesterday. We still use those. Amalya's images will live on long after you and I are gone.

"There's a Latin phrase I learned in my training: *Mortui vivos docent*. It means 'The dead will teach the living.' But that's not true. In emergency medicine, people die all the time, and we fail exactly the way we failed before. Because there is a shortage of donors worldwide, we don't learn how to do a thing differently," Scotty said.

"It is one of the greatest wastes on the face of the earth."

CHAPTER ELEVEN

The Dance
2013–14

I t had been nearly four years since Thomas's donation, and it was becoming clear there were more chapters yet to unfold.

In November 2013, Dr. Zieske from Schepens surprised us with an incredible gift: a copy of a study that may have been a result of Thomas's donated corneas. "Potential of Human Umbilical Cord Blood Mesenchymal Stem Cells to Heal Damaged Corneal Endothelium," published in the journal *Molecular Vision* on March 2, 2012, was very likely based on Thomas's donation. We couldn't know for sure because of confidentiality issues, but it could be a written record of Thomas's contribution to the advancement of medical science. It contained beautiful images of what were possibly Thomas's eye cells.

And the study itself was even more interesting.

The cornea is the clear outer layer of the eyeball, sort of like the eye's windshield, and it looks like a transparent contact lens. Endothelial cells in the cornea do not regenerate, so if a cornea gets damaged, it stays damaged. Also, corneas naturally get worse as we get older. A newborn baby has all the corneal cells the person will ever have, and we lose about 10 percent of them every decade. In addition to normal wear and tear, some genetic diseases lead to vision impairment. One in particular is Fuchs's endothelial dystrophy. According to the National Institutes of Health (NIH), Fuchs's is a disease of middle age, affecting approximately 4 percent of people over age forty, with women being affected more often than men. In its milder forms, patients don't necessarily notice a change; in advanced cases, patients experience vision loss.

For more than a century, corneal transplant has been the only option for those with a damaged cornea. One of the drawbacks to a corneal transplant is that there's a propensity for rejection, so patients often need to use immunosuppressive eyedrops for the rest of their lives.

Also, a corneal transplant involves getting stitches in your eye.

In the study published in *Molecular Vision,* researchers at Schepens described their attempts to find a way to make the cornea heal itself. They tried adding stem cells that were derived from donated umbilical-cord blood to the donated cornea— maybe Thomas's—and found that the corneal cells did show signs of being able to regrow.

The study was dense with scientific jargon, and it was difficult for me to really understand its importance. I wanted to know what the study really meant and to learn more about its context from someone not personally involved, so I contacted Dr. Albert Wu, an oculoplastic surgeon and corneal researcher at Mount Sinai School of Medicine.

Dr. Wu has a B.S. in molecular biophysics and biochemistry from Yale and an M.D. and a Ph.D. in molecular and cellular biology from the University of Washington. In addition, he's currently working on his own corneal research project involving stem cells.

"Is it possible that this study could take some people off the corneal transplant list?" I asked him.

"Absolutely," Dr. Wu said. "This study is just the beginning. It shows that, potentially, mesenchymal cells can be used to heal damaged corneas so our patients no longer require transplant." He went on to explain that in the United States every year, about forty thousand corneal transplants take place and that, worldwide, about six million people suffer from corneal blindness.

Thomas could have restored sight in up to two people if his corneas had gone for transplant. Instead, thanks to his contribution to this study, he was assisting a research effort that could potentially restore sight to millions of people. (As of the publication date of this book, this study has since been cited in seventeen more studies.)

Thomas was giving this proud mom more and more to brag about with every passing year. And he wasn't done yet.

In April 2014, WRTC invited me to speak about Thomas at a National Donate Life Month event at Children's National Medical Center in Washington, DC. This is the facility where Thomas's eye and liver recovery took place, so I was delighted to give a talk there.

When Thomas's body left our home for the first time without one of us, Ross and I wondered where he had gone. Four years later, I was finally able to ask WRTC to give me a behind-the-scenes tour of the most likely path Thomas's body took after he left our home. I wanted to see the operating room where the recovery happened, and I also wanted to meet any of the team who might have been working that day or who may have been involved in the work on Thomas.

After the event, I had the honor of meeting Dr. Mark Batshaw, executive vice president, chief academic officer and

physician-in-chief, and director of the research institute at
Children's. But most fascinating to me was that, as one of the
doctors who actually performs the infusion of hepatocytes on
children, Dr. Batshaw was an end user of the Cytonet treatment. I excitedly explained that my son was a Cytonet donor,
and told him about my visit.

Then it was time for the tour. This is where Thomas had
been; it was hard to believe I was getting to fill in more of his
story.

I was joined by an entire medical team, including an anesthesiologist and some transplant nurses. We began where ambu-
lances drop off emergency patients, and then we headed up to
the operating-room floor, where we changed into white gowns
and put blue paper booties over our shoes.

The operating room that Thomas had been in, OR #1, was
occupied, so we toured one next door. I couldn't resist asking a
question.

"Were any of you working here that day—March 29, 2010?"

One nurse raised her hand. "I didn't work that morning, but
I was an employee here at that time."

"Has anyone here been in the room when a recovery
happens?"

Everyone nodded and looked at the floor.

"What is it like to be in the room during a recovery?" I
asked.

There was a pause. It was clearly a hard question to answer.

Eventually, one of the nurses said, "Emotionally, it's difficult.
You spend all your energy thinking about saving these children's lives. When all the efforts fail, it gets to you." Everyone
nodded in recognition. "I remember that, the first time I saw
a recovery, the hospital was really good about providing counseling, and making the chaplain available and everything. But

while you are doing it, you are just focusing on your job. I guess it's the adrenaline. Once the day was over and I got in my car, I just broke down. *That's* when I needed the counseling."

Someone else said, "You feel so bad for the parents that it came to this. You wonder how they feel about it."

I really wanted to give these wonderful people some succor.

"I was actually excited to be able to donate," I said. "This was the one good thing that might come from my son's death. I was like, 'Please, please, take everything you can.' I was sending good vibes to the whole team—like, 'Please let this be success-ful. Do whatever you need to do.'"

Donating had lifted my burden, not made it heavier. I felt so lucky to be able to put faces to the team that had looked after Thomas, and was also glad they now had seen the face of a parent who had been blessed by their work. I hoped that seeing my gratitude for their work also gave them permission to do their job without feeling embarrassed or guilty. Being part of a recovery is an act of kindness for the donor's family as well as for the recipient. I wanted this team to hear that, unvarnished and straight from a parent's mouth.

The importance of this moment, and the emotion it brought out in me, overwhelmed me, and I suddenly felt very dizzy. I had to sit down and put my head between my legs.

Luckily, I was already surrounded by a team of medical pro-fessionals.

Eventually the blood started flowing again, and I asked Kimberly Woodard, Hospital Services and Professional Educa-tion specialist with WRTC, how eye recoveries are done. She told me that she performs them all over the state of Maryland, and that she often transports the tissue in her car: there's only a short window of time in which they can be processed, so she happily drives them to Medical Eye Bank of Maryland.

"So there are corneas sitting next to you in the passenger seat?" I asked.

"Yeah," she said, like it was no big deal.

"Do you ever get a speeding ticket?" someone asked her.

"Well, we are not supposed to speed, but I admit I have gotten a ticket with eyes in the car. I still had to pay it," Kimberly said, and everyone booed.

A few months later, as part of my job at AATB, I went to Baltimore to attend the annual meeting of the Association of Organ Procurement Organizations.

This annual meeting is the national conference for all fifty-eight OPOs from around the country, as well as other industry groups, and I was really excited because I would finally get to meet Bill Leinweber and Jeff Thomas of the National Disease Research Interchange. I wanted to tell them in person how much I appreciated NDRI's facilitating Thomas's cornea donation to Schepens.

Not willing to leave it to chance that I'd run into them, I made an appointment to sit down with them so I could tell them about Thomas and how important it had been to me that I was able to visit Dr. Zieske and learn about the amazing work the scientists were doing to restore sight to people with corneal blindness.

After I showed them pictures of Thomas and talked about tours I'd gotten, Jeff Thomas said, "Since I knew I'd be seeing you here, I pulled up Thomas's file to remind myself of where his gifts went."

And then he dropped his bombshell.

"It looks like his retinas were also sent out for research."

Surely if the retinas had also been placed, I would have heard about it before. I had visited the facility that processed his eyes, and they didn't mention anything. I thought, *Jeff must be thinking of some other donor.*

"No, I don't think so," I said. "I just went to Old Dominion Eye Foundation last year and talked to Bill Proctor. He confirmed what WRTC had told me back in April 2010. Only his corneas were placed."

"I'm pretty sure the retinas were, too," Jeff said. He looked like he was sure of himself, and I was confused—and suddenly hopeful. What if another donation was out there somewhere?

"I'll look into it when I get back to the office," Jeff said.

I wished his office had been open right then.

After a long day of sessions, at the evening reception I ran into some WRTC friends. As we mingled and politely sipped our pinot grigio, a distinguished man with white hair and glasses joined us.

"Sarah, do you know Dr. Carlos Fernandez?" someone said.

I had never met Dr. Fernandez but always hoped I might, because he was the medical director of WRTC, and the surgeon who recovered Thomas's liver.

We made small talk for a few minutes, and then I plucked up the courage to say what I wanted to say.

"I'm a donor mom. My son was an infant, with anencephaly."

"I'm so sorry," Dr. Fernandez said.

"I understand that you are the surgeon who did his liver recovery."

"Oh, when was it?"

I explained the circumstances of the recovery—the hospital, the time of day, the size of the baby. He said he remembered it.

"The donation brought our family a lot of healing," I said. "It was early in the morning. So thank you for getting up that early."

Dr. Fernandez and I sat next to each other during dinner that night and continued our lovely conversation. Later on, we

had an epic time on the dance floor. As I said to one of his colleagues, "Don't let the gray hair fool you—this guy has moves!"

Shortly after the AOPO conference, I got news I'd long
been waiting for. I could hardly believe it, but it was true: Jeff
Thomas and Bill Proctor contacted me to tell me that yes,
Thomas's retinas had indeed been donated to a research facility.
There had been a paperwork mix-up, which is why ODEF had
no record of the donation.

But NDRI did. The retinas . . . after all that.

I knew I had another trip to make. And I couldn't wait.

SUE'S STORY

Sue Scott was just thirty-six years old in July 2012 when her doctor told her there was nothing more he could do for her: her cervical cancer had metastasized to her lymph nodes, and she had tumors all over her body.

"There must be options," Sue said.

She was met with silence.

Radiation?

She'd already had the maximum.

Chemotherapy?

There was none that worked for her type of advanced cancer.

Sue Scott said, "Stick a fork in me. I'm done."

Nine months earlier, on Halloween 2011, after Sue had started to noticed some vaginal bleeding, she was handed down the verdict: she had a one-and-a-half-inch tumor in her cervix. The two most common types of cervical cancer are squamous cell, which begins in the cervical lining, and adenocarcinoma, which starts in the cells that make fluids. Sue's was an aggressive adenocarcinoma that had likely been growing inside her for years.

Some cancers are caused by environmental factors, such as smoking or exposure to other toxins, and some are genetic or caused by random mutation. Sue's cancer was the result of an infection by human papillomavirus (HPV), by far the most common sexually transmitted infection out there; something on the order of fourteen million new cases occur every year.

According to the Centers for Disease Control and Prevention, there are more than two hundred kinds of HPV virus, and 90 percent of men and 80 percent of women will contract at least one kind during their lifetimes. The good news, if there is such a thing in a disease that is so prevalent, is that most strains of HPV are deemed low-risk and do not cause cancer—just warts, a.k.a. *condylomata acuminate*, on or near the genitals, anus, mouth, or throat. But about a dozen strains of so-called high-risk HPV can cause cancer. Nearly all cases of cervical cancer, as well as most anal, oral, throat, and tonsil cancers, and a large percentage of vaginal, vulvar, and penile cancers, are the direct result of HPV infection—most commonly HPV types 16 and 18.

The U.S. Food and Drug Administration has approved three vaccines against high-risk strains of HPV: Gardasil, in 2006; Cervarix, in 2009; and, in 2014, Gardasil 9—which covers, as the name suggests, a total of nine strains. These new drugs provide excellent protection against new HPV infections, including the high-risk strains, thereby preventing as many as 90 percent of cervical and anal cancers, but they don't help patients who already have an infection. Given the size of Sue's tumor, she had probably contracted HPV before any of these vaccines became available.

Cervical cancer used to be a significant cause of death for women of childbearing age in the United States, according to the National Institutes of Health. But with the introduction of the Pap smear in the 1950s, which allows doctors to examine cells under a microscope to look for abnormalities, the frequency has dropped dramatically, since precancerous lesions can be treated or removed before they turn malignant. In other words, regular screening makes the disease rare, and highly treatable if caught early. That said, of the approximately twelve thousand women who do develop cervical cancer every year, about four thousand will die of it. Unfortunately for Sue, her cancer wasn't found until it was pretty far along.

After her diagnosis, Sue's doctors put her on a standard

three-part course of treatment for a patient with her degree of disease: external radiation—also known as external beam radiation therapy, or EBRT—in which X-rays are beamed at the cancer from outside the body (like a regular X-ray but with a much higher dose of radiation); internal radiation, or intracavity brachytherapy, in which the radiation material is put in a metal tube that is then inserted into the body, applying the radiation directly to the cervix; and finally, a course of low-dose chemotherapy.

Sue thought, "Some of everything. I guess that's good."

When her treatment was complete, a CT scan found no detectable signs of her tumor.

But three months later, Sue Scott found herself with new and worrying abdominal pain. This time, her doctor prescribed a positron emission topography, or PET, scan, which found that her cancer not only had returned, but had spread catastrophically. Sue had tumors on her liver, her bladder, her uterus, and her abdominal wall and in the lymph nodes in her groin and chest.

What Sue hadn't known at the start of all this was that the standard course of care works for only 65 percent of cervical cancer patients. Sue was one of the 35 percent for whom it didn't work. With the results of the PET scan in hand, her doctor informed her that there was nothing he could do.

It was time to see what else was available.

Sue Scott first met with an oncologist at the National Institutes of Health, who said, "We have a chemo that we're trying on HPV cancers. We haven't had a lot of success with it yet, but we can do that for you."

Trying to maintain a positive outlook, Sue said, "What's the success rate?"

"We're not talking cure here. We're talking slowing the growth."

"Well, I'm talking cure. Is there anything for cure?"

At this point, Sue's mother had been, by grim coincidence, diagnosed with uterine cancer, and had had a hysterectomy. Sue paid $350 out of pocket to get a consultation with her mother's surgeon; he was her seventh doctor in nine months.

This new surgeon told Sue that, depending on what he found when he opened her up, she might need, at the least, a radical hysterectomy, which would take out her uterus, cervix, and ovaries. At worst, he discussed the possibility of something Sue had never even heard of: exenteration. As the American Cancer Society describes it, exenteration is the most extensive pelvic surgery—a procedure so drastic you can't imagine someone thought it up. It is performed when a woman has experienced a recurrence of cervical cancer, as Sue had. The surgery removes not only the reproductive organs that are excised during a radical hysterectomy, but also the vagina, bladder, urethra, and rectum. It is called a total pelvic exenteration if the surgery also includes two ostomies, or surgically made openings: one for urine, called a urostomy; and one for stool, called a colostomy.

"Basically, they would cut off my lower half and stick my legs back on," said Sue, employing admirable gallows humor.

When Sue woke up from the surgery, she didn't know how much of her body she still had. So she asked her mother, Sharon, who was with her in the recovery room, "Do I still have my vagina?"

"You do. Your rectum and your bladder, too."

Sue was understandably relieved—until, that is, the surgeon came in to see her. It turned out that her cancer was so extensive that there had been no point in the most debilitating surgery since it wasn't going to cure her cancer.

It was another great blow, and Sue thought she'd hit another dead end, until the surgeon said, "At this point immunotherapy is your only chance."

"What the heck is that?"

"Basically, it's a way of enhancing your body's own immune system to fight the cancer. I don't know if there's a clinical trial for your type of cancer, but I'll look into it."

Sue was finally in luck. Through her surgeon she learned that Dr. Christian Hinrichs, of the National Cancer Institute in Bethesda, Maryland—which is part of the National Institutes of Health—had just started an immunotherapy trial that May. This is how her first conversation with Dr. Hinrichs went:

"How many people are in your study?" Sue asked.

"Four."

"The entire study is four people?"

"Yes."

"Is it working for any of them?"

"It's too early to tell. We're only three months out. We have one patient for whom it seems to be working. She has had some tumor reduction. The other three have not."

"And this person you're treating who has had some response— does she have the same kind of cancer as I do?"

"No, she has squamous cell."

"So my best chance of treatment is in a trial with four people in which one person may be responding with some tumor shrinkage but still cancerous, and her cancer is a different type than mine?"

"That's correct. But we do believe it could work for adenocarcinoma patients as well. That is, we don't have any reason to believe it *couldn't* work; we just don't have any patients with that type in the trial as yet."

The great well of positivity and fortitude that had gotten Sue this far crumbled in that instant, and she began to cry. Her best chance was something that hadn't worked for anybody yet. Without *any* treatment, her surgeon had said, she had probably less than a year to live. She had a dozen tumors, including one the size of a golf ball protruding from just above her belly button that she could feel with her hand if she pressed down on it. (She had been so horrified the first time she felt it, she never touched it again.)

Despite her tears, Sue managed to ask Dr. Hinrichs to explain what the treatment entailed.

Hinrichs's boss, Dr. Steven Rosenberg, was the chief of surgery at the National Cancer Institute and a pioneer in the field of developing and treating patients with advanced cancers with gene therapy and immunotherapy. As Jerome Groopman wrote in an article called "The T-Cell Army" in the *New Yorker* in April 2012, Dr. Rosenberg "developed a strategy called adoptive cell transfer in which T cells are taken from a patient's tumor and given immune stimulants such as interleukin-2 which cause them to replicate. Then they are put back in the body." T cells, which get their name from the thymus, where these cells originate, "are a potent type of white blood cell that destroy cells infected with microbes that they recognize as foreign."

When Dr. Hinrichs first joined Dr. Rosenberg's group, the two men were focused on melanoma, a cancer of the skin, which, if caught early, is highly treatable and which, if not, is highly lethal. One of the processes they worked on was one in which they removed a patient's tumor and then grew huge numbers of T cells out of that tumor. In some cases, the treatment made the cancers go away and stay away.

In refining the process, the researchers wanted to identify specific tumor protein, or antigen, that the T cells could target. "What we found was that we could treat the tumors, but we also caused a lot of injury to the healthy tissue that also expressed the antigen," Hinrichs said. (This occurred because antigens can make both a normal melanocyte and a cancerous melanocyte.) "Patients would develop severe rashes and experience transient hearing and vision problems. It made the therapy untenable."

Hinrichs became interested in HPV-caused cancers because it

was possible to target the HPV antigen in the tumor and spare the healthy tissue. Someone who has an HPV cancer, such as Sue's cervical cancer, no longer has the virus, but the antigens remain, which are what cause the cancer. "Our best chance," Hinrichs said," is to target antigens that are *only* in the tumor."

That's what the trial was engineered to do when Sue Scott arrived on Hinrichs's doorstep. Her cancer was just what he was looking for.

But nothing came easy to Sue Scott. After assessing her condition, the NIH refused to accept Sue into the trial because she was too sick. By this point she had developed blood clots in her lungs, and those had to be treated first. Then it was discovered that she had hydronephrosis—one of her kidneys was swelling with backed-up urine because a tumor was blocking the ureter that connect the kidney to the bladder. It put her at high risk for infection.

It was recommended that Sue join a chemo trial to see if chemo could reduce some of the tumors. Sue refused: she wanted the immunotherapy treatment. Chemo would sap her strength, and she wanted to be 100 percent.

The only option left was to put a stent into the ureter to prop it open, but such stents are prone to infection. If Sue developed a kidney infection when they had already knocked out her immune system—well, it could kill her.

"I don't care," Sue said. "I have to do this treatment. I won't talk to anybody. I won't kiss anybody. Just put in the stent and trust that I won't get an infection."

While the board at NIH reviewed her case during the fall of 2012, she sent them a handwritten letter begging to be included in the trial. She addressed it to "the kind, heart-led, wise, hard-working and (I'm guessing) dashingly good-looking team of doctors in charge of my fate. Signed, from a gal who had an unfortunate string of events that led me to VBC (very bad cancer)." And because the review coincided with a presidential election, Sue filled the envelope with confetti and wrote "Vote 'Yes' on question 'Sue Scott!'"

At her next monthly check-up, her medical oncologist was extremely concerned. "You've been without treatment for over six months now," she said. "You need to be in treatment. You can't keep waiting for this immunotherapy."

"I have to do this," Sue said.

"Can I be honest with you?"

She thought, *The answer to that is always no.*

The doctor said, "It doesn't matter what treatment you do at this point. None of these things is likely to work."

And that's when Sue Scott finally lost her temper.

"You've got a lot of nerve!" she said. "It matters to *me*. I know the chances of this immunotherapy working for me are slim to none. I know it hasn't worked for anybody else yet. But if this is the last good thing I can do for the next person who ends up in this horrible place—and that's what we're talking about here—then that's what I want to do."

Sue looked over at her mother, who had joined her for this appointment as she had so many others. Her mother was so moved by what her daughter had said, she was crying.

"I guess it's your decision," the doctor said.

In her annual Christmas letter that year, Sue wrote to her loved ones, "Even if it doesn't work for me, maybe the doctors will learn how to help the next woman who ends up here. Maybe this is the final gift I can offer the world."

Finally, at the beginning of February, after the clots in her lungs had resolved, she was accepted into the trial. In the six months since she had first approached Dr. Hinrichs, only three other patients had been accepted, making Sue patient number eight.

The first step was to put in the stent to fix Sue's kidney problem, and it worked out great: no infection. Then she had surgery to remove the tumor on her liver to isolate the T cells to be subsequently grown in the lab. It would take five weeks to grow a sufficient quantity, and Sue, being Sue, figured that was enough time for an adventure.

Sue and her mom, Sharon, had always wanted to go to Australia, but Sue figured that now they weren't going to get there. When she said as much to her mom, Sharon said, "Oh, we're going to Australia." The doctors at NIH thought a seventeen-hour flight each way was a bad idea for someone with late-stage cancer—not to mention that while they were there, they would be spending their time in the outback, a hundred miles from the nearest hospital.

It hardly needs to be said that Sue and Sharon went to Australia. When they got back, Sue was energized and ready for the most difficult three weeks of her life.

During her first week back, Sue received chemo to knock out her own immune system. She lost her hair and felt sick to her stomach. At the beginning of the second week, a nurse brought in an IV bag filled with what looked like condensed milk.

Sue's brother, a super-smart math guy, was in the room at the time, and as the nurse hung the bag up on the IV stand and arranged the tubing to begin the infusion, he asked her, "Do you know how many cells are in there?"

"We sure do. There's actually a calculation on this bag that tells us how many are in there." The nurse looked at the bag and began to read off a complicated equation. "I think that comes to seven and a half billion cells."

Sue said, "Wow! Incredible there are so many in that little bag!"

When the nurse left the room, Sue's brother said, "I think she might have gotten the equation wrong and it's more than that."

"How could it be *more?*"

A few minutes later, with the infusion complete, a doctor came in to check on Sue.

"I'm Dr. Yang," he said. "How do you feel?"

"I feel seven and a half billion cells heavier," Sue joked.

"Seven and a half? Who told you that?" the doctor said.

"One of the nurses."

"Well, she missed a decimal place. You're actually seventy-five billion cells heavier."

Her brother smiled and gave her a look that said, "I told you so!"

Sue was amazed how fast and painless the infusion had been. But then the really hard part started.

The next day, Sue began to receive doses every eight hours of interleukin-2, a protein that encourages the TILs (tumor infiltrating lymphocytes) to grow. By the time she received the fifth dose, she couldn't eat and she required oxygen full-time. The next few days were even more brutal, but at the end of the twenty-one days, Sue managed to walk out of the hospital and head home. Now, all she had to do was wait.

Two months later, miraculous news arrived: there was no detectable trace of tumors on Sue Scott's scans, and her lymph nodes had returned to normal.

Doctors have continued to check Sue every six months, but as of 2015, Dr. Hinrichs was able to tell her, "I think you're in the clear."

The science that led to Sue's miraculous recovery—one she never expected for herself—is complicated and changing all the time. "It's a fast-moving target," as Dr. Hinrichs puts it. But Sue, now an advocate for NIH, has come up with an amusing way of describing what saved her life:

"I tell people that my immune cells were like these superintelligent little nerds with pocket protectors that knew my cancer was there and it wasn't supposed to be but they didn't have the strength to more than say, 'Excuse me, I don't think you're supposed to be here.' The doctors took out those little nerdy cells and they sent them to kung-fu school, trained them how to find the cancer cells and kill them, and then they put them back in. Those same cells went and found my tumors and were like, 'You need to get the eff out,' like bouncers at a bar. Those little nerdy guys came back with a vengeance and went all through my body and found the tumors and kicked them to the curb."

Sue's case was written up—sadly, without any reference to nerdy cells and bouncers—in the March 2015 issue of the *Journal of Clinical Oncology*. The article gives the game away even in its very title: "Complete Regression of Metastatic Cervical Cancer After Treatment with Human Papillomavirus-Targeted Tumor-Infiltrating T Cells."

There were a total of sixteen patients in the trial in which Sue participated; only she and one other woman saw their tumors go away. Another woman had some shrinkage of her tumors, but it was temporary.

In the other patients, sadly, there was no response.

What researchers learned in studying Sue's cells versus the cells of the women who did not respond to the treatment was that the patients with the greatest reactivity against HPV antigens were the ones who did the best in the trial. As a result, doctors now know that potential patients who have a similarly high level of reactivity will have the greatest likelihood of responding well to treatment; and those without the reactivity can be spared a difficult protocol that would cause them unnecessary misery.

Sue Scott didn't offer herself up for the NIH trial expecting to help herself; rather, she thought she might at least help the next woman unlucky enough to find herself in the same terrible shoes. But Sue was fortunate in two ways: The first was that she got sick when she did; if she'd received the same diagnosis even a year earlier, there wouldn't have been a trial for her to join. The second piece of good fortune was that the trial protocol worked spectacularly well for her.

The long-term benefit for future patients because of what Christian Hinrichs and his team at NIH learned from the trial is boundless. A handful of patients, only two of whom recovered, have, through their contribution, furthered and augmented the arsenal that medical science has to combat what was once a near-certain death sentence.

And for Sue, she gets to advocate for change with a smile on her face and a joke at the ready.

CHAPTER TWELVE

The Quest Isn't Over Yet—
The University of Pennsylvania

March 23, 2015

T he news about the retinas was fantastic. And it meant I started to hope that I could make one more trip to meet the scientists who were working with my son's donation.

As I thought about ways to most effectively connect with Thomas's retina researchers, I figured I'd try a new tactic. In keeping with the style of the letters that are often written from donor families to transplant recipients, I penned a "Dear Researcher" email. In it, I explained who I was and what had happened, and asked if they could tell me why they had needed the retinas. I also broached the subject of a lab visit one day.

In September 2014, I sent the email to Christina Jenkins—associate director with Old Dominion Eye Foundation—and asked her if she could forward it to the person who had wanted the retinas. She said that ODEF had never done such a thing before, and though she could not guarantee a response, she would give it a try.

It took two days.

On September 25, 2014, I received an email from Dr. Arupa Ganguly, a professor in the Department of Genetics at the Perelman School of Medicine at the University of Pennsylvania. Dr. Ganguly thanked us for the donation and explained that she was studying retinoblastoma, a rare but deadly cancer that affects children under the age of five.

And yes. My family was welcome to visit her lab.

A few days later Dr. Ganguly and I spoke on the phone. I could feel my heart beating hard; I would never get used to connecting with Thomas's "colleagues."

"It is an honor to talk to you," Dr. Ganguly said. Imagine—an honor. This was almost too much. "I can't imagine how you must feel," she went on. "Thomas made the ultimate sacrifice."

Whoa, whoa, whoa, I thought. *Sacrifice? We didn't kill our son just so we could donate his body to a study.* The word seemed to imply that she felt guilty, or somehow indebted to me, and it took me by surprise. I didn't want her to feel that way at all.

"I don't see it that way," I said. "If you hadn't wanted Thomas's tissue, it would have been buried in the ground where it wouldn't be helping anyone. Our choice was not between an alive child and a dead child. We would have picked the alive child, of course. So our choice was between burying our dead child and donating his tissue. Donating to your study added a layer of meaning to his life that was not there before. So we are very grateful he could be part of your study."

I asked Dr. Ganguly if she remembered receiving the tissue; after all, it was almost five years earlier.

"Yes, I remember that day. I have a log book, but I don't need to look in it. It's the only healthy tissue sample we received in six years."

Dr. Arupa Ganguly had been waiting on a sample like

Thomas's *for six years*? I was floored. It validated my hunch that donating for research was worth the effort. It did matter to someone—and it mattered a lot. Arupa told me that the tissue was so precious she was saving it, because she didn't know when she might get more.

And then she said something that stopped my heart.

"I still have some of it in a lab freezer. You can see it if you like."

Yes, I wanted to see it. Seeing Thomas's journey from the very beginning to the very end—how many people get to do something like that? To see what a donation looks like, and understand what it means. And to be in the presence of a lost boy's RNA.

It had been one of the most meaningful phone calls of my life.

Yes, I wanted to see it.

The tour of Dr. Ganguly's lab was set for Monday, March 23, 2015, which would be the twins' fifth birthday. We decided to make a stop at the National Disease Research Interchange headquarters, too, ahead of our trip to see Dr. Ganguly. In the meantime, Arupa sent Callum a toddler-sized Penn T-shirt for his collection.

Ross, Callum, and I drove to Philadelphia a day early and spent the Sunday at the child-friendly Please Touch Museum. We had a dinner at an Irish pub and carried all of Callum's birthday presents up to our hotel room so he could open them in the morning. But I couldn't wait for the next day to arrive.

Callum woke up bright and early that Monday, eager to get on with our celebration of his special day. His favorite gift was a two-foot-tall Godzilla he had been talking about for weeks.

Our appointment at NDRI in Center City was set for 9:30 A.M. When we arrived, an athletically wiry man in his fifties, with a pair of reading glasses perched on his forehead, was waiting in the lobby. I had contacted the *Philadelphia Inquirer* to see if they thought there was a story in my family's trip, and they had sent the best of the best: Michael Vitez, a thirty-year veteran staffer with a Pulitzer under his belt for his human-interest stories.

In a conference room, NDRI president and CEO Bill Leinweber and about thirty members of his staff were sitting around a large table.

Bill thanked us for coming: we were, once again, the first donor family to request a visit. I introduced myself, Ross, and Callum to the assembled group.

I gave them my presentation about Thomas and the researchers I had already met, and I thanked them for making this journey possible. When I was done, I handed Bill a framed copy of a photograph of Thomas.

"May I have a high-res digital copy? I'd like to make an enlargement for the lobby here," he said.

Bill presented Callum with a birthday card and several stuffed animals as presents. I went around the room introducing myself to every member of the staff and thanked them for the work they were doing. It was a privilege to meet the people who were vital to so many groundbreaking medical advancements.

Michael Vitez joined us in the cab for the ride over to Penn, where Maiken Scott of radio station WHYY—I'd contacted NPR, too—and her photographer, Kimberly Paynter, met us. Joining us was *Philadelphia Inquirer* photographer David Maialetti. It was quite the media crowd.

Jessica Ebrahimzadeh, a genetic counselor working in Dr. Ganguly's lab, and senior science communications manager Karen Kreeger were waiting for us. It was a sprawling complex, and we were led through the labyrinth of hallways and elevators to Dr. Ganguly's fourth-floor lab in the Anatomy Chemistry Building. When we got to the conference room, Dr. Ganguly's staff and yet another photographer—this time from Penn—met us.

Dr. Ganguly had not yet arrived, so I took the opportunity to introduce myself to everyone else. "Thanks for having me," I said. "It's an honor to be here, so thanks for letting this happen."

I sat down next to Jennifer Yutz, the lab manager. "Do you remember Thomas's tissue coming here?"

"I do, yes."

"Did it come in Styrofoam or a cardboard box?"

"Either." Her hesitation made me realize that no one had ever asked Jennifer these questions before.

"Did it say Human Eyes on the side?"

There was a ripple of nervous laughter in the room.

"It did, yes," Jennifer said, with a smile.

Eventually Dr. Ganguly arrived, and she quickly set about explaining why it was so important to have received Thomas's donation. It had been the first healthy infant retina sample her lab had ever received, and it was vital to her work.

In order to understand the uncontrolled cell growth of cancer, Dr. Ganguly needed to be able to compare diseased eye tissue with healthy eye tissue. She had samples of diseased tissue, but, as she put it, "there is no normal situation in which one can get a healthy sample." In other words, a child had to die for her to get what she needed to complete her study. I remembered James Selby Jr.'s poem from the donor family gathering:

> *For me to live,*
> *you had to die.*
> *While my family rejoiced,*
> *your family cried.*

But it wasn't just that a child had to die. The logistics of collecting the tissue—which had to be done within four hours of the death, with the tissue then placed in a particular solution so that the DNA and the messenger RNA (mRNA) were not degraded—made viable healthy samples very rare.

"Please don't feel guilty about it," I said. "You didn't make my son die." Then I repeated for all to hear what I'd said to her during our initial phone call: "If you didn't have his tissue, it would be in the ground not doing anybody any good."

Dr. Ganguly smiled. "That is a relief to hear. Thank you, Sarah. When I first learned that you wanted to come here, it immediately changed my perception of my work. When we received the sample in 2010, it was simply entered into a data-base and assigned a number. Thomas is RES360. It's completely impersonal. But now, here is a mother who has lost a baby boy. It made me sad, because now this sample that had been so good for my research was connected to a deceased child. Then I wondered how I would react. Would you like to know what we did with your son's eyes?"

"I'm happy that you have them," I said. "Share what you learn with the medical community, and share it with us when you can. If you get published, that would be cool."

I gave Dr. Ganguly a framed photo of Thomas, like the one I had given Bill Leinweber, with a brief inscription commemo-rating the date of this visit.

Thanking everyone for their time, Dr. Ganguly took us to her lab.

As we walked down the hall, Callum ahead, and I heard him say, "Oh!" When I got there, I found him with his arms wrapped around a large inflatable dinosaur, a surprise gift from Dr. Gan-guly. He didn't lose the smile—or let go of that dinosaur—for the rest of the visit.

Back at Dr. Ganguly's office, Jennifer Yutz joined us again and showed me a black-and-white marbled composition book. "This is our log book. We make an entry for each sample that we get."

Jennifer opened the log book to a page with an entry for March 30, 2010. As the 360th specimen the lab had received, it was assigned the number RES360.

"Oh my gosh, that's him! Ross, look at this!"

There was Jennifer's handwriting; she had personally recorded Thomas's donation.

Then they showed me the FedEx envelope that Thomas's retinas had arrived in.

"Can I make a copy of these?"

"We have copies for you."

That shipping label felt like an heirloom to me.

Jennifer Yutz said, "Come with me." We walked back through the lab toward a freezer across from a bank of student lockers.

Jennifer put on thick blue rubber gloves before opening the door and then pulled out a tray holding 1.5-milliliter vials. There appeared to be hundreds of them in that freezer. Jennifer pointed to two of them. "There," she said. I leaned closer. "Careful, don't touch." The ambient temperature in the freezer was minus 80 degrees Celsius, or minus 112 degrees Fahrenheit. (That's about 100 degrees Fahrenheit colder than the threshold for getting frostbite.) "That's the RNA that we isolated from Thomas's retina tissue."

When I looked closely, I could see the handwriting in blue ball-point ink.

"RES360."

That was it. That was Thomas's donation in those little tubes. They had saved some of his tissue because it was so valuable, and they hoped to use it again in the future.

RNA in a test tube is like a turtle on a fence: you know it didn't get there by itself. At that moment, I thought of all the people who had worked together to make it happen. Counting professionals connected with Inova, WRTC, ODEF, NDRI, and Penn, there were at least twenty-five people who worked together to make those little vials possible—not counting the people who helped improve and contribute to these processes over the course of more than fifty years of research. There was the person who invented the preservation solution; the person who figured out how to recover eyes; the person who figured out how to extract RNA; the people who founded WRTC, NDRI, the Lions Clubs, Old Dominion Eye Foundation, the Penn Genetics Diagnostic Laboratory. The list was long.

It was a lot to take in, and not just for me: the lab staff had never met a donor's family before. I think we all needed a moment to take a deep breath. I had preordered lunch for the staff and the media, so we filled our plates, ate, and relaxed. I passed around the book of photographs of Callum and Thomas that I'd made for Callum and the memory box that contained Thomas's handprint and medical bracelet.

I asked some of the staff how they got into this field in the first place. One person said that when she was little she had been given a kit that showed you how to get DNA out of a strawberry—DNA you could see with the naked eye. Just when I thought she must have been the most science-focused kid in the world, two of her colleagues chimed in that they, too, had the strawberry DNA kit as a child. I realized then that these people were really in the right job. Dr. Ganguly told a story about getting hit by a car on the way to lunch, and still attending the U.S. Supreme Court to watch the proceedings of a historic case about patenting genes in which she was a plaintiff.

"You lead an exciting life," I said, and noticed that the staff all nodded and laughed in a way that betrayed their affection and respect for their colleague.

Further evidence of the passion of these amazing people came when someone chimed in that they intended to offer Callum an internship.

"I won't be here by the time he's ready for that," Dr. Ganguly said, but she had a smile on her face that seemed to say she would, in fact, make sure she was around then.

"I will be around," Jennifer Yutz said. "I love it here. I'm not going anywhere."

And with that, it was time to serenade the birthday boy with a rousing rendition of "Happy Birthday." Callum blew out a candle, then tucked into his favorite treat—a sticky cinnamon bun. The staff even gave him a toy science kit with goggles and beakers.

We all got gifts that day. Callum got his dinosaur and his sticky bun; the scientists got to put a real name to RES360; and Ross and I got to share in the wonder yet again of what Thomas's gift was doing—not just for these researchers, who had waited so long for someone like him to come along, but for all the patients in the future whose vision, and maybe even lives, would be saved.

March 29—the date Thomas died—is a tough one for me. I want to recognize it because it's a day that changed our lives profoundly. I don't exactly want to celebrate it, but ignoring it and doing nothing doesn't feel right, either. Fellow bereaved mom Anna Whiston-Donaldson, the author of *Rare Bird: A Memoir of Loss and Love,* calls the anniversary of the death of her son the "Crapiversary," which sounds about right.

But Sunday, March 29, 2015, had at least this to recommend it: Michael Vitez's article about our visit ran in the *Philadelphia Inquirer* and on its companion website, Philly.com, that day.

Five years after Thomas's death, something good was happening on this day. Quickly, the story of Thomas Ethan Gray spun around the globe; the story eventually received more than one million clicks. I had contacted the local media only because I thought it might inspire people in Philadelphia to appreciate what was happening in their hometown, and also to perhaps register to donate. I was surprised and delighted that the story of my son resonated with such a wide audience all over the world.

Dr. Ganguly said that there is no normal circumstance that would make the tissue of a healthy child available. In other words, she considered the death of a child somehow abnormal, and I disagree. Although we might not always talk about it or hear about it, children and babies die every day of trauma and diseases. According to the CDC, more than nine thousand children under the age of fourteen died in the United States in 2013. We don't know how many of them donated healthy retinas for research, but we do know that Dr. Ganguly didn't receive any that year despite being on the waiting list for years. My hunch is that the number of donations was zero, because parents are not aware that they need to proactively ask to donate.

This was about to change.

CHAPTER THIRTEEN

Who Was Afraid and Why

At every step of my journey to track down my son's donations to research, I willingly and enthusiastically shared my information, and the researchers I met seemed open to meeting me and to sharing what they were doing. But it seemed like I kept bumping up against confusion around confidentiality rules, and I wanted to know why.

The history of medical research is peopled with thousands of well-intentioned researchers looking to improve the health and well-being of mankind, from Dr. William Halsted's discovery of the antiseptic method, which revolutionized modern surgery by making it largely survivable, to Jonas Salk's discovery of the polio vaccine, and beyond. But in a world of people doing good work, sometimes the bad seeds get the most attention and tarnish the reputation of the field. For example, some of the worst cases include the inhumane experiments conducted by Josef Mengele at Auschwitz; the human guinea pigs who suffered the dire effects of untreated syphilis in the Tuskegee experiments; and the unwitting contribution made by Henrietta Lacks that was famously documented in Rebecca Skloot's

The Immortal Life the Henrietta Lacks, the book I was reading when I was waiting to see the psychic Kizzy in Scotland.

But those are the exceptions. The vast majority of research being conducted today is, as Jeff Thomas of NDRI says, "for the betterment of mankind."

And yet the sometimes overly restrictive rules—or simply the wary attitudes—continue to get in the way.

Unless consent is obtained, when organs, eyes, tissues, and blood are donated for research, all identifying descriptors are removed, and the donations are assigned a number. But they can be re-identified if needed; that's an FDA requirement. If the tissue ever needs to be recalled because of an infectious disease scare, say, the donations in question must be tracked as a matter of public safety.

Traditional research practices include keeping all participants' identifying information confidential: researchers receive de-identified donations. Living donors or authorized parties sign consent forms stating they understand that they will not receive results of any scientific study made using this donation.

The Belmont Report: Ethical Principles and Guidelines for the Protection of Human Subjects of Research, published by the National Commission for the Protection of Human Subjects of Biomedical and Behavioral Research in 1979, established the guidelines for research on humans, which were in turn adopted by the National Institutes of Health. And it was based on these regulations that *The Federal Policy for the Protection of Human Subjects*—also known as "the Common Rule"—was published in 1991. The Common Rule stipulated requirements for assuring compliance by research institutions, for obtaining and documenting informed consent, and for the creation of institutional review boards, or IRBs.

An IRB must be established by any institution "sanctioned

by the Federal Government to conduct research" from its own faculty as well as nonaffiliated nonscientists. Further, "any study involving research on human beings must go through the IRB."

The intention was that IRBs were to protect research participants from fraud and abuse. However, IRBs also have their downsides. As Steven J. Breckler, executive director for science of the American Psychological Association, has said, "Increasingly, we hear horror stories about IRBs that are imposing incredible burdens on researchers, creating bureaucratic nightmares and otherwise hindering the progress of research." Rather than furthering research, IRBs can lean toward simply protecting academic institutions from lawsuits—CYA (cover your ass) run amok.

In fact, Carl E. Schneider, professor of law at the University of Michigan, recommended in his 2015 book, *The Censor's Hand: The Mismanagement of Human-Subject Research,* that IRBs be completely eliminated because they tend to delay or distort research that could otherwise be helping advance scientific discovery for the betterment of patients.

In response to a history of complaints about inappropriately shared medical records, the Health Insurance Portability and Accountability Act of 1996—known as HIPAA—was passed, leading to the U.S. Department of Health and Human Services issuing their "Standards for Privacy of Individually Identifiable Health Information." These standards ushered in a new era in which patients began to see their medical records as their own, and not the property of their doctor. Before HIPAA, a doctor might give a copy of a patient's medical record to the patient's employer or spouse, or even to a fellow physician. A doctor was even allowed to call a patient's voice mail at work and leave a recording including sensitive test results and medical information. HIPAA stopped all that, instead putting discretion in the hands of the patients.

So HIPAA now allows patients to request their medical records at any time, and to request a list of people who have accessed their electronic medical records. Patients also have the right to submit a correction if there is a disagreement about a doctor's statement. Health-care providers are not permitted to share medical information with an employer or a spouse anymore without the patient's written consent. HIPAA also allows the patient to determine which phone number a health-care provider is allowed to use, and whether they have permission to leave a message about the patient's medical treatment.

However, when it comes to research, HIPAA also facilitates researchers having access to data than can be useful in their work, unlimited by privacy concerns. With all the genetic work going on, scientists need huge amounts of such data, but HIPAA also requires researchers to de-identify samples that they work with so that participants' identities are unknown. Once a bio-specimen is de-identified, it is no longer protected by HIPAA. This advances medical science, for sure, but some people may be uncomfortable with the thought that their tissue, or their loved one's tissue, is floating around out there anonymously.

But it gets more complicated still, since scientists have proved since the rules were first put in place in the early 1990s that it's now possible to re-identify tissue with DNA and other tests.

To my eye, at least, the issues boil down to one thing: informed consent. Many people are happy to participate, just as I was, but they want to know about it, and they want to give permission.

As of 2016, the Department of Health and Human Services is considering a change to the Common Rule that would require explicit permission from patients for scientists to use leftover tissue from surgeries or biopsies or blood donations. Some researchers worry that this will create a bureaucratic nightmare, while others, like Duke University's Misha Angrist, think that the days of anonymous tissue samples are long past their expiration date.

In 2007, Angrist became the fourth participant in the Personal Genome Project at Harvard Medical School, in which volunteer participants agree to have their entire genome sequenced and made public. Founded in 2005 by George Church, a professor of genetics at Harvard Medical School, and still run by him in 2016, the project states as its operating principle that sharing data is "good for science and society." At the time of its founding, very few sequences had been completed. As of 2015, the project had compiled more than two hundred whole genomes. But sequencing has become much more common now, to the point where you can submit a sample of your dog's DNA for genotyping for less than one hundred dollars if you want to know what breed Fluffy's great-great-grandparents were.

Angrist, who sports a salt-and-pepper close-cropped goatee and thick glasses, is an intriguing hybrid: he has a Ph.D. in genetics from Case Western Reserve University and an M.F.A. in writing and literature from the Bennington Writing Seminars. (Angrist wrote about his experience with the Personal Genome Project in his book *Here Is a Human Being: At the Dawn of Personal Genomics*.)

The Harvard Personal Genome Project wasn't just making genomes available to other researchers; it was also making them available to the public. Participants are specifically not promised confidentiality since "genomic data is as unique as a fingerprint to an individual and can never be fully anonymized."

Angrist is a passionate advocate for the sharing of research results with human participants. He's written numerous scholarly articles on the subject, including one titled, "You Never Call, You Never Write: Why Return of 'omic' Results to Research Participants Is Both a Good Idea and a Moral Imperative." According to the article's abstract: "Return of genomic data to those who want it, even if a difficult undertaking and even if the meaning of the data is unclear, engages participants in science and the research enterprise, and positions them to be better stewards of their own health and wellbeing."

Angrist thinks the real problem with institutions insisting on confidentiality is not the Common Rule, or privacy issues, but simply that they are risk-averse. There's a history of treating people who participate in research as anonymous. If researchers don't have to know any personal information about the subjects whose tissues they work with, they don't have to take any responsibility for those people. Without that responsibility, they can focus all their time on their work rather than on placating participants who might be requesting more information about what they're doing (a thing Angrist has sympathy for).

There is a tendency to dehumanize research subjects; even calling them *subjects* is dehumanizing. According to Angrist (and others, including many involved with the Precision Medicine Initiative), those who choose to contribute to these studies should be referred to as *participants* or *partners*.

"I think we have come to a place where the term *subjects* is not only offensive, it's inaccurate. If you are a subject, you have nothing to say about anything. If you are a participant or a partner, then you do have something to say. And science needs to listen," says Angrist.

In his field of genomic studies, participants expect to be told what researchers learn about them. Indeed, the incentive that is often offered to prospective participants is a copy of the survey results.

When Angrist was on Duke's IRB committee, he saw first-hand how restrictive the consent forms could be. He would regularly see protocols that said the investigator would not return information to the prospective participant because it was not clinically actionable—that is, the participant wouldn't be able to do anything with the information other than know it. "It's condescending," Angrist says. "The consent form is already twenty-eight pages long and designed to protect the institution from getting sued. To say also that you will get nothing, and it will be better for you, just feels like an insult."

So how does one turn around this entrenched culture of keeping information close to the researchers' vest? Incentives, Angrist says. He thinks institutions that are funding the research, such as the National Cancer Institute and the NIH, could add a little more funding to help researchers figure out how to return results. "Returning results is a concrete way for an investigator to say to a participant, 'I have some information about you. It may or may not be useful, but if you are interested in receiving it, I am prepared to share it with you.'" In other words, it's a way for scientists to treat participants as people rather than as cells on a spreadsheet.

To my mind, as long as scientists are pursuing ethical research—which I imagine is the case most of the time—and participants are informed and openly consenting, the barriers seem largely unnecessary. I knew that the researchers I spoke to about Thomas's gifts were not trying to steal our son's tissue. Since Thomas was dead, these donations were his legacy. These were his first and last contributions to the world. What good is a legacy if no one in the family can pass it down because we don't know about it?

CHAPTER FOURTEEN

From Donation to Discovery
October 30, 2015

F ive years after Thomas's death, a lot had changed. What started as a broken heart blossomed into a sense of pride in my son's accomplishments. His donation exposed me to a world of scientific and medical advancements I would not have even imagined before. I had the privilege of meeting brilliant and kind professionals who are changing the field and saving and improving lives on a daily basis.

Thomas led me to a new career, and his deeper purpose gave me one, too.

At the end of October 2015, the National Disease Research Interchange (NDRI)—the organization that facilitated the donation of Thomas's cornea to Harvard and his retina donation to the University of Pennsylvania—celebrated its thirty-fifth anniversary with a symposium at the Union League of Philadelphia: "*From Donation to Discovery: The Critical Role of Human Tissue in Research.*"

Since its founding three and a half decades earlier, not only had NDRI become a leader in the world of recovering and distributing human organs and tissue for research—what they call "biospecimens" in the profession—they had also developed a number of specialized programs to help researchers in specific ways.

The first panel of the day was called "Advancing the Nation's BRAIN Initiative." BRAIN stands for "Brain Research through Advancing Innovative Neurotechnologies," and the initiative was launched by President Barack Obama in April 2013 to support further understanding of the human brain and uncovering new ways to treat, prevent, and cure brain disorders like autism, epilepsy, schizophrenia, Alzheimer's, and traumatic brain injury. And the government wasn't fooling around: the National Institutes of Health invested more than $130 million in BRAIN in the first two years alone.

Why so much interest in the brain? Because every year, approximately one in eighty-eight children in the United States is born with autism or a related disorder, and more than five million older people will be diagnosed with dementia—a number that's likely to rise as the boomer generation moves into old age. Also on the rise are ALS, or amyotrophic lateral sclerosis (a.k.a. Lou Gehrig's disease); Parkinson's; and progressive supranuclear palsy, a degenerative neurological disorder that affects about twenty thousand Americans and for which there is no effective treatment or cure.

Suicide is a significant public health issue as well. It remains one of the leading causes of death in this country: it's tenth overall, fifth for ages forty-five to fifty-nine, and second for ages ten to twenty-four. Suicide among young Native Americans is nearly twice the national average. Women are three times more likely than men to attempt suicide, but men are four times more likely than women to actually kill themselves.

Here are some of the other sobering statistics for suicide

in the United States, according to the American Foundation for Suicide Prevention: a million people attempt suicide every year, and forty thousand are successful. Veterans account for more than 22 percent of suicides. (U.S. Department of Defense guidelines make it very difficult for researchers to gain access to the brains of deceased veterans for the purpose of research, whether death was from suicide or traumatic brain injury.) And 90 percent of people who commit suicide have a diagnosable psychiatric disorder.

Given these upsetting numbers, researchers are keen to investigate the physiological aspects of brain function that might help explain why suicide is such a big problem.

So here's the big challenge that medical science faces: We all learned in school that the brain is the most complicated organ in the body, which means it remains—even with all our advancements—one of the least understood. There are something like one hundred billion neurons sending about one hundred trillion messages to one another, which makes the brain "one of the greatest mysteries of science and one of the greatest challenges in medicine," according to the BRAIN Initiative. Given the ambitiousness of the project, NIH is collaborating with scientists and engineers from other government agencies, such as the Defense Advanced Research Projects Agency (DARPA), National Science Foundation (NSF), U.S. Food and Drug Administration (FDA), Intelligence Advanced Research Projects Activity (IARPA), and private partners. It's a huge undertaking, and these studies require donated whole brains.

On the dais for the first panel at the NDRI symposium were Mark Frasier, senior vice president of research programs at the Michael J. Fox Foundation for Parkinson's Research; Richard D. Hasz, vice president of clinical services at the Gift of Life Donor Program; John Madigan, vice president for public policy at the American Foundation for Suicide Prevention (SPAN/ USA); Dr. Daniel Perl, a man with many titles including director of the Neuropathology Care Center for Neuroscience and Regenerative Medicine; and Thor D. Stein, a neuropathologist with the U.S. Department of Veterans Affairs.

There was also Deborah C. Mash, director of the University of Miami Brain Endowment Bank, which is one of just six designated brain and tissue biorepositories in the country. They're supporting research into ALS, multiple sclerosis, Huntington's disease, traumatic brain and spinal injury, developmental disorders like autism and Down syndrome, and mental-health issues like depression and bipolar disorder. Founded in 1987, the bank holds more than two thousand brains, with another five hundred people on the list to donate.

As the experts convened to discuss challenges in acquiring tissue to study, it became clear that recovering brains for research was rather different from acquiring other organs and tissues. For instance, the medical/social interview, now called the Uniform Donor Risk Assessment Interview, wouldn't have covered the kind of information that scientists looking at the brain need. A person can donate a kidney or skin without anyone needing to know if he or she ever heard voices, but not so the brain. Trying to come up with a uniform list of questions for potential brain donors and their families was a challenge.

In addition, families need to feel comfortable with the decision to donate, since they also make a decision about what kind of funeral to have. Some family members may wish to see the decedent one final time at an open-casket funeral. Facing the death can help some people believe it and come to terms with it. Initially, there was concern from both families and funeral directors that a brain-recovery incision would alter the appearance of the decedent and force a difficult decision on a family in this position: "Do we donate a brain for research, or do we have an open-casket funeral?" OPO professionals wanted to make it possible to do both.

Rebecca F. Cummings-Suppi, L.F.D., C.T.B.S., is manager of tissue recovery and preservation at Gift of Life Donor Program in Philadelphia and is also a licensed funeral director and embalmer. She spoke about this challenge at the 2014 American Association of Tissue Banks annual meeting. Becky and her team developed a brain-recovery technique that involved making an incision from ear to ear at the back of the head where the skull meets the spine. I was touched by the pride she took in caring for both the needs of a grieving family and the research protocol.

"I don't believe in putting anything of value in the ground. Whether it's a diamond ring that can be passed down to another generation, or if it's tissue for transplant or for research," she told me. "That's how cures happen."

The second panel that day focused on research for rare diseases—which, generally speaking, don't have relevant animal models such as mice. (Even common disorders, like age-related macular degeneration, have this problem, because mice don't get this disease, so there's no way to study it in them. That's why researchers like Patricia D'Amore at Schepens Eye Research Institute at Harvard need human tissue to complete their work.)

NDRI's Rare Disease Initiative collects donated tissues, organs, and blood as well as DNA and cell lines for more than one hundred rare conditions. Some of these include amyotrophic lateral sclerosis, or Lou Gehrig's disease—a progressive degenerative disease that targets nerves in the brain and spinal cord and causes progressive muscle weakness and paralysis until the patient is no longer able to breathe on his or her own. (Perhaps the most famous sufferer, aside from the New

York Yankee great after which it gets its nickname, is physicist Stephen Hawking, who has managed to survive for many years beyond the usual life expectancy for this brutal disease). Also included is Lewy body dementia—also known as dementia with Lewy bodies—a disease named after scientist Friedrich H. Lewy, who identified the abnormal protein deposits in the brain that disrupt normal functions such as perception, thinking, and behavior. (The late comedian Robin Williams was found to be suffering the early stages of this disease when he took his life in 2014.) Another disease included is sickle cell disease, a genetic condition characterized by abnormal hemoglobin in the red blood cells. (At the moment, only a stem-cell transplant can cure this otherwise lifelong condition, and life expectancy is between forty and sixty years in the United States, which is nevertheless up from fourteen years just forty years ago.)

Notable among the veteran scientists on the dais for this second panel was the smiling face of a teenage girl. That's because the discussion centered in particular on NDRI's partnership with the Cystic Fibrosis Foundation and Vertex Pharmaceuticals, which together have developed the first-ever medications to treat the underlying cause of cystic fibrosis rather than just its symptoms. The young woman's name was Mara Cray; she was a patient.

Cystic fibrosis (CF) is a life-threatening genetic disease that affects thirty thousand children and adults in the United States and seventy thousand people worldwide. CF causes a buildup of thick, gluey mucus in the lungs, pancreas, and other organs. The mucus in the lungs clogs air passages and traps bacteria, which can lead to severe infections that damage the lungs. In the long run, the damage can be such that the only option is a lung transplant. Today, the life expectancy of a person with CF is under forty years. In the 1950s, it was fewer than six.

The Cystic Fibrosis Foundation was founded in 1955 by a group of parents whose children had the condition. At the time, CF kids were not expected to live long enough to enroll in grade school. In 1980, the Cystic Fibrosis Foundation created a research development program to speed up the search for a cure. That move contributed to the discovery, in 1989, of the CF gene, the first major step in understanding the disease at its root. The Cystic Fibrosis Foundation has been behind just about every drug invented to treat the disease.

In the mid-2000s, clinical trials began on the first oral medication that targets the mutated protein responsible for CF. In 2012, the FDA approved ivacaftor (Kalydeco) for certain CF patients over age five. In 2015, the FDA approved Orkambi, a two-drug combo of ivacaftor and lumacaftor, for about one-third of CF patients over age twelve. It was a huge breakthrough for the treatment of this disease, presenting the possibility for the first time of CF patients living out something closer to the life span of someone without CF.

This most recent milestone occurred in large part thanks to an effort begun by the Cystic Fibrosis Foundation with an assist from NDRI. In 2006, NDRI began receiving donations of diseased lungs from CF patients who received transplants. The donations were transported to Vertex, a global biotechnology company that studied the tissue to develop two new drugs designed to combat the disease at its biological root. Since CF, like other rare diseases, has no correlative in the animal world, to really make advances in treatment, researchers needed human tissue.

"We needed a relevant pharmacology model to assess our drugs," said Eric Olsen, Ph.D., Vertex vice president and CF franchise leader. "Airway cells derived from the native tissue provided by NDRI allowed us to better understand" how the drugs might work in patients with CF, he told the panel.

Chris Penland, Ph.D., director of research at the Cystic Fibrosis Foundation, has said: "The most important contribution that NDRI makes is their ability to reach out into the community and acquire tissues to help drug discovery efforts. Almost every primary cell used in the research to make these discoveries was from a lung NDRI acquired."

You could draw a direct line between the donation of those lungs by people who had no choice but a lung transplant and future CF patients who may be saved from ever needing one.

For example, Mara Cray. She has been just one direct beneficiary of those sixty years of research and about two hundred donated CF lungs.

In parallel to all this research using donated lungs, in 2014 NDRI launched a five-year initiative called the Molecular Atlas of Lung Development Program (LungMAP), which is funded by the National Heart, Lung and Blood Institute and the NIH. For this project, NDRI is looking specifically for pediatric lungs in order to study pediatric lung diseases—ones that develop in utero and in early childhood.

That's a tall order, but had it been available when Thomas died, he might well have been eligible to donate. It would have been a privilege to be a part of this project.

Perhaps the most ambitious program that NDRI supports by providing human tissue is the genotype-tissue expression (GTEx) program, which was launched in October 2010 by the National Institutes of Health's Common Fund.

As I learned from the Duke study, gene expression has a huge impact on a person's health. The federal government decided to create a massive data bank to study how that expression affects genes and correlates to various genetic diseases.

The National Human Genome Research Institute (NHGRI) described it in terms even I could understand: "Each cell in the human body contains a complete set of genes, yet not every gene is turned on, or expressed, in every cell in the body. To function properly, each type of cell turns different genes on and off, depending on what the cell does. For example, some genes that are turned on in a liver cell will be turned off in a heart cell."

What GTEx sought to do, as NHGRI explained, was put those two ideas together to study how gene expression is regulated in different organs in the body, which would go a long way toward explaining the "underlying biology of many organ-specific diseases."

Spearheaded by NDRI's leadership team, NDRI set out to collect thirty-three different kinds of tissue from approximately 160 deceased donors.

NDRI started receiving donated tissue for GTEx in July 2011, from approximately six deceased donors each month. (One of the guidelines for the GTEx project was that recovery had to occur less than six hours after death. NDRI averaged just three to four hours for most of their recoveries, well under the target.) Two years into the effort they had collected thirty-three different types of tissue from 175 donors, for a total of sixteen hundred samples. Scientists in the GTEx project then studied the DNA and RNA from those samples, focusing largely on the tissue types they deem most valuable: fat, heart, lung, skeletal muscle, skin, thyroid, blood, tibial artery, and nerve.

That was just the first phase. In the second phase, NDRI worked with five OPOs—Gift of Life Donor Program of Philadelphia, LifeNet Health of Virginia Beach, Center for Organ Recovery and Education in Pittsburgh, Washington Regional Transplant Community in Washington, and LifeGift in Houston—for an additional 150 organ donors and 100 tissue donors.

The specimens were all sent to the National Cancer Institute's Human Biobank, except for the brains and spinals cords. Those latter donations went to Dr. Mash's Brain Endowment Bank at the University of Miami, where scientists isolated cells from various regions of the brain and sent them to the GTEx lab, storing the remaining tissue for future studies of the central nervous system.

The excitement in the scientific community over this project is palpable. Meenhard Herlyn, D.V.M., D.Sc., a professor at Wistor Institute in Philadelphia and chairman of the board at NDRI, said, "GTEx has an ambitious program to finely analyze genetic and epigenetic variations in human cells within each of the different organs. The results, once we learn to interpret the massive amounts of data, will bring us one step closer to understanding the many subject signatures of human organs."

It was also notable that, given the priority assigned to transplant versus research by organ-procurement organizations and eye and tissue banks, Richard D. Hasz, the vice president of clinical services at the OPO Gift of Life, had this to say: "Research is a fundamental part of our mission, and organ transplantation, as it exists now, would not exist without effort like this. GTEx provides an additional opportunity to create a legacy for donors and their families, with the ultimate goal of contributing through research for the betterment of mankind."

The third and final discussion of the day focused on improving the matching function of donating for research. The featured panelists were Barbara Koenig, a professor of medical anthropology and bioethics at the University of California, San Francisco; Helen Moore, chief of the Biorepositories and Biospecimens Research Branch at the National Cancer Institute; Kevin Myer, president and CEO of the OPO LifeGift in Houston; Timothy Westfall, director of Biopta, Ltd.; Dr. Serge

Przedborski, a renowned professor of neurology and vice-chair of research in the departments of neurology, pathology, and cell biology at Columbia University; and Susan Stuart, president and CEO of the Center for Organ Recovery & Education in Pittsburgh.

Medical science had made enormous and unforeseen strides in the years since NDRI started its work collecting pancreases for investigators to study diabetes. Until now, the focus has been on collecting as many organs and tissues that are unsuitable for transplant as possible. But as researchers' investigations, and therefore their needs, become more sophisticated, NDRI has worked to develop new tactics for identifying donors who match the new and unique requests.

Traditionally, the role of OPOs has been to recover organs for transplant, not necessarily organs for research. In the United States alone, more than 123,000 people are waiting for a life-saving organ to be available. In the last few years—and especially with the arrival of these enormous government-sponsored research endeavors—the number of requests for research tissue has increased exponentially. The Center for Medicare Services (CMS) became the overseer of the entire network of organ-procurement organizations across the country, and all the different kinds of organ and tissue recoveries they now perform—all because of kidneys.

Back in 1972, the Social Security Act created an entitlement covering the cost of dialysis and transplant for all patients suffering from end-stage renal disease (ESRD) who were eligible for Medicare coverage, which covers approximately 90 percent of all patients with this condition. Today, OPOs are largely reimbursed by hospitals when they provide organs for transplant, but if there is any shortfall, Medicare makes up a small portion of the difference—but only in the case of kidneys. In order to be eligible for that reimbursement, all OPOs must meet the performance standards required by CMS for OPO certification.

In 2006, CMS added a third metric for certification—donation for research. The "Medicare and Medicaid Programs Conditions for Coverage for Organ Procurement Organizations (OPOs) Final Rule," published in the *Federal Register* on May 31, 2006, reads: "Like organs for transplantation, organs for research are a precious national resource. We believe OPOs should recover organs for research whenever possible to aid researchers looking for new therapies for debilitating and fatal diseases, many of them the same diseases that cause end-stage organ failure in patients waiting for transplants. Although recovering organs for research is not an OPO's primary mission, the organs it places with researchers may help lead to treatments or cures that will reduce the transplant waiting list as surely as organs that are used for transplantation. We believe that providing an incentive for OPOs to recover organs for research will increase the number of organs available to researchers throughout the country. . . . Nevertheless, while recovering organs for research is vitally important, we do not want OPOs to recover organs for research at the expense of organs for transplantation."

According to Lori Brigham, president and CEO of WRTC, who has been with the Washington, DC–based OPO since its inception in 1987, "It's an enormous amount of work to do research recovery. You have to have the additional staff and surgical resources to be able to do that. WRTC oftentimes supports research recovery, and we do not get reimbursed fully for it. That's one of the reasons a lot of OPOs are unable to strongly commit to the recovery of organs for research. The researchers will contact the OPO asking for various types of organs and tissues to be used in their research. But a lot of times they do not have the funding to pay for the recovery of the tissues and organs—the additional operating-room time; the addition of surgical staff to go into that operating room to recover that organ or tissue for that researcher; the preservation, packaging, and transportation of that tissue or organ sample. You also need to consider the additional time it takes to discuss the research with the family during the donation authorization process. There's a considerable amount of work that's involved in research donation and research recovery."

Immanuel Rasool, manager of research and living donation at WRTC, works closely with NDRI and other research organizations across the country. Rasool's job is to find placements for organs and tissues with researchers; he also teams up with the International Institute for the Advancement of Medicine, the group that linked Bethany Conkel's son, Amalya, up with researcher Scotty Bolleter. Rasool also reaches out directly to researchers at academic institutions in the Washington, DC, area.

Rasool explained the growing challenge in research donation: "Researchers are picky about what they want. For example, someone may want only male skin, or skin from someone of a certain age." He also pointed out a surprising bureaucratic obstacle that sometimes comes up: office hours. "Researchers need [to receive] the organ or tissue pretty quickly, but they may not be available twenty-four/seven. We could have a donor who is perfect match on a Friday night, and we can't find researchers because they're generally not working weekends."

Rasool concurred with recent research showing that the majority of potential donors would happily donate for research if they were given the option and the research was explained well to them or their families.

The boom in stem-cell research has, for instance, created a demand for testes, which contain adult male germ line stem cells that can be altered into "embryonic-like" stem cells, according to scientists at Georgetown University, where one such study was being conducted. When Rasool first heard a request for this, he thought, *How am I supposed to request testes from a grieving family?* But when the reason was explained to families, many were happy to donate.

Some tissues may not be needed immediately, so they are stored for the future—which is another part of what the GTEx project is about. Harvard University's T. H. Chan School of Public Health has a huge stash of hair samples and freezers full of toenails—clippings from more than one hundred thousand people, if you can imagine such a thing—with which researchers hope to better understand ovarian cancer. The idea is that blood will tell scientists what's in your system only at the moment it's drawn, but hair and nails hold onto trace elements and hormones, so scientists can check levels of these things over several months.

Jeff Thomas of NDRI said that to him the big revelation about the GTEx project was that 70 percent of families agreed to donate when they were told about its aims. Thomas's father, who was suffering from a form of frontal-lobe dementia, was signed up to donate to the University of Pennsylvania Perelman School of Medicine's Center for Neurodegenerative Disease Research. Researchers are monitoring his disease progression while he's alive, and then they will have his brain to study when he dies.

"I'd like to think we'd get to the point where the general public was aware that research donation is an option and they can understand the benefits of that gift to future generations," Thomas said.

I was invited to speak at NDRI's thirty-fifth-anniversary dinner that evening, which was being held in the imposing Lincoln Hall at the Union League of Philadelphia—a room dominated by portraits of past heads of the Union League.

As Ross and Callum and I walked in, one of the first people we saw was Michael Vitez, who'd written about us in the *Philadelphia Inquirer* and who, fittingly, would be the emcee of the evening's festivities. I chatted with him about how popular his story had been—another sign that Thomas's donation had reached and affected so many lives.

As the speeches began, I realized that I was part of a much bigger effort to move science forward. Bill Leinweber, the president and CEO of NDRI, welcomed us all and laid out all the things NDRI does, and then Michael Vitez called me up to the podium. I was joined onstage by Ross and Callum, now five and a half years old and getting used to Mommy talking about his brother, Thomas, in front of people.

As I stood in front of hundreds of faces, I realized that these professionals understood, more than any other people on the planet, this major event in our lives. These were my people now.

In my speech I explained that I had initially been curious about where Thomas's donations went and what difference they made, and that although I might have been the first person to go on this quest, I didn't want to be the last. I praised NDRI: given all the privacy issues, they could have stopped me, but they only helped. And I closed with a message about the power of sharing information and included the story of Matt Might, which Seth Mnookin told in the *New Yorker* in July 2014. Matt's child was diagnosed with a genetic defect so rare that no research study would invest the money to study the disorder unless other patients were found. Matt then wrote a long essay on his own website called "Hunting Down My Son's Killer." The piece went viral on Twitter and Reddit and was republished in the tech blog *Gizmodo;* as a result, he was connected with thirty-six more patients with the same disorder. He essentially crowdsourced a rare-disease research sample—a critical step in securing research. The NIH began a formal investigation of the disease, and in less than four years that research was already translating into drugs to treat it.

While I was talking, Callum stood quietly with his dad. My boy seemed so at ease in the spotlight now—I guess he'd had some practice—and everyone was impressed by how calm and good he was, this boy who had cried out when his twin took his final breath five years earlier.

Back at the table, everyone praised Callum.

"Mommy, am I famous?" Callum whispered to me.

"Yes, a little bit," I said.

Later, NDRI recognized various OPO donation partners from around the country who had worked on the GTEx initiative, and I realized again how the effort to support research is fueled by hard-working people from all over America. There was the Center for Organ Recovery & Education (CORE), based in Pittsburgh and servicing 155 hospitals mostly in western Pennsylvania and West Virginia; the Gift for Life Donor Program, which works all the way from Delaware to New Jersey; Texas-based LifeGift; LifeNet Health from Virginia Beach, which covers southern Virginia; and my beloved Washington Regional Transplant Community.

NDRI then introduced the inaugural D. Walter Cohen Service to Science Award, and gave it to D. Walter Cohen himself. A periodontist by trade, Dr. Cohen led NDRI until he became its chairman emeritus at the start of 2007.

Dr. Cohen took the stage and took us all back to the moment in 1952 when his life changed. He had been attending a lunch at Princeton University that was also attended by Albert Einstein. The meal had been a benefit for the Hebrew University, and one of the financial donors offered to double a $250,000 pledge if Einstein would shake the hand of the donor's wife. Hearing this, Einstein jumped out his chair so fast to grab her hand that his spectacles skittered across the floor. Dr. Cohen said that such an image of putting ego aside to help a good cause had stayed with him to this very night.

As the attendees put on their coats, said their good-byes, and headed out into the chilly October night, I thought of the past and the future. Albert Einstein, born in 1879; D. Walter Cohen, born in 1927; and Thomas Ethan Gray, born in 2010—all three forever connected through this evening, this organization, and this effort.

Mara's Story

A Sword and a Shield

Mara Cray was born in 1996 in Voorhees, New Jersey, and was diagnosed with cystic fibrosis at birth. Her parents, Sharon and Mike, were already familiar with the disease because her brother Ian, five years old, also had it. (Her other brother, David, is eight years older but doesn't have the disease. Growing up with two sick siblings led him into the medical field, but he opted to treat animals rather than people.)

Growing up, Mara and Ian went to doctor's appointments together. "I was the youngest, so I would do whatever my older brother did anyway. Just the fact that my older brother had CF meant it was okay for me to have it, too," said Mara.

Since CF was somewhat normal in the Cray household, Mara didn't think much about it. She wasn't uncomfortable telling people she was sick, taking her medication in the school cafeteria, or sucking on an inhaler in gym class. And because she didn't have a problem with it, her friends didn't, either, visiting her in the hospital when she needed IV antibiotics for a few weeks every year, but not making a big deal about it. CF was just part of her life.

Yet she had some unique challenges that her non-CF friends didn't have. CF lungs are like fly traps for bacteria. A person without CF can easily cough out invaders, but a CF patient cannot. Because of this, CF lungs provide a warm, humid, permanent home where bacteria can get comfortable, learn to resist antibiotics, and develop into "superbugs" such as *Pseudomonas aeruginosa,* the most common cause of mortality among CF patients. These super-bugs are harmless to someone with healthy lungs, who can simply cough them out, but they can be deadly for CF patients. A superbug called *Burkholderia cepacia* is so dangerous that the Cystic Fibrosis Foundation has banned anyone with a positive *B. cepacia* culture from any foundation events, meetings, or offices.

Some of these superbugs were already detected in Mara's lungs when she was five years old. Because she took antibiotics so fre-quently, the bacteria learned to adapt over the years. This meant that great care had to be taken when Mara visited places that could harbor bacteria—places like airplanes, public bathrooms, and gym locker rooms. In addition, environmental irritants such as bathroom cleaners and smoke can be a hazard for CF patients, who already have compromised lung capacity. As a result, Mara suffered through more than one campfire with her friends, never able to find a seat in the circle where the smoke didn't find her.

"Campfires I hate," Mara says. "The idea is nice—sitting around a fire with your friends and all that—but five minutes in, I have no voice and I'm coughing uncontrollably."

Although Mara attended a mainstream school for most of her childhood, many exceptions had to be made to allow her to do this. She and her parents met with teachers and administrators to adjust her schedule and workload. Mara needed at least one hour of treatment per day, consisting of two to four medications inhaled by nebulizer, plus airway clearances, which are effected either with a compression vest or chest physical therapy (clapping) every morning. As a result, the family arranged Mara's classes so that she could arrive later than the other kids. In the evenings, the same regime had to be followed. If she was too sick to complete homework assignments, arrangements were made for her to do make-up work, and, not sur-prisingly, she was not strictly held to the school's attendance policy.

Having a condition like CF can be emotionally isolating for patients. Whereas many people with chronic illnesses are able to connect with peers in disease-specific support groups, meeting others with CF can be life-threatening. Because of the possibility of cross-infection, CF patients need to maintain a distance of at least six feet from one another, since that's the distance droplets from sneezes and coughs can travel. Mara likened it to CF patients having a group restraining order against themselves. Fortunately, modern-day sufferers at least have the Internet, where they can join online support groups, but it's still not quite the same as seeing people face to face.

When Mara was fifteen years old she began experiencing a significant decline in her energy levels and respiratory health. Her doctors would sometimes prescribe oral ciprofloxacin (Cipro) to treat infections, but when it was bad they recommended IV antibiotic treatments of tobramycin, together with a second antibiotic to target whatever bacteria she was hosting at the time. The drugs knocked out her lung infection but gave her side effects of terrible nausea, fatigue, and depression. One other side effect that CF patients are warned about: the medications inflame and weaken tendons and joints. Mara depended on a regular mile-long run to help clear her airways, but when she was enduring a round of antibiotics, she couldn't run, which made her breathing worse.

Mara came home from her first day of tenth grade exhausted. By the time she went to bed that night, she realized she had spent her entire evening doing treatments and hadn't touched her homework. Sadly, it was clear to her that she wouldn't be able to keep up, so her parents eventually withdrew her from regular high school and enrolled her in Keystone National High School, an online, self-paced high school program for students with unique scheduling needs. Her mom and dad also checked in with Mara's doctor to see if there was anything they could do to stop the rapid decline in her health, and asked about a new clinical trial that was backed by the Cystic Fibrosis Foundation. It was still looking for participants, and Mara fit the criteria to join.

And so, in July 2013, at the age of sixteen, Mara, together with her parents, decided that she would become what Mara calls "a human guinea pig," and registered her for the experimental drug trial.

The trial involved taking five pills in the morning and four pills in the evening. In Mara's mother's lay terms, "DNA makes RNA. RNA makes protein, and the proteins are defective. They don't allow for the processing of water and salt. So this treatment corrects the defective protein." This kind of treatment is called a "protein assist" or "protein correction." Instead of treating an infection, this would *prevent* an infection.

Gradually, over the course of months, Mara began to notice an improvement. She stopped getting sick as frequently; her energy level increased; she didn't feel as run-down as she had before; and some of her lost lung function returned. Her rapid decline not only stopped; it reversed direction. This was almost unheard-of.

There is a coda to Mara's story.

In 2001, when Mara was four years old, she lost her comrade: her nine-year-old brother, Ian. Though he had CF, he died from something else. After what seemed like a bad case of stomach flu, he lapsed into a coma, and a week later he died. Ian was diagnosed with viral encephalitis, an inflammation of the brain that can start with flu-like symptoms. His parents, Sharon and Mike, were asked about organ, eye, and tissue donation by their local OPO, Gift of Life, in Philadelphia.

Ian was thoughtful and sensitive, and lived "like he knew he didn't have much time," said Sharon. He wrote a sixteen-chapter book about a fantasy world, with themes surprisingly sophisticated for someone who was only nine years old. The book was about self-sacrifice, saving other people, and what it means to be heroic. "He liked to think of himself as someone with a sword and a shield," said Sharon. The preface to his book reads, "I want something to happen to me. Something strange. Something different. . . . I want to go to a different world. I have a feeling that one day I'll get my wish." Mike and Sharon thought that donating Ian's body for the benefit of others was the right choice.

Initially, Mike and Sharon thought that his having CF would preclude Ian from being a suitable donor, but they learned they were wrong. Ian was a candidate to donate for research as well as transplant. His kidneys, corneas, and heart valves saved and changed lives through transplants. His liver was donated to NDRI for research on drug toxicity and metabolism. His lungs, trachea, and pancreas were donated to the University of North Carolina for CF research. (Fourteen years later, the UNC researcher still remembers receiving this donation. It was unique because the lungs had such little CF damage compared with the ones that are donated after a lung transplant.) Ian's gallbladder was also donated for medical and scientific research.

The bottom line is: The donation of Ian's organs, eyes, and tissue for research may very well have contributed to the studies that could lengthen or save Mara's life—as well as the lives of thousands of other CF patients around the world.

Today, Mara's prognosis is good. As of 2015, she takes the commercially approved dose of the drug Orkambi, the direct result of the trials she participated in. Her energy is high enough that she's consistently completing her high school classes and is scheduled to graduate from high school as part of the class of 2016. In the past, she could rely on getting a lung infection every six months or so, which would put her out of commission for two to three weeks. So far, it's been eighteen months with no infection. This kind of freedom allowed her to do something she would have never attempted in the past: she has two part-time jobs—one at a bakery, where she bakes wedding cakes, cupcakes, and pastries; and one at a health club, teaching tennis to children. She is healthy enough that she recently traveled to Washington, DC, to speak on a panel before Congress. The panelists reminded Congress of the importance of funding basic research. Maybe Ian's little sister has a sword and shield of her own.

Mara says that she was born at a good time to have CF. In the last twenty years, great strides have been made in treatment thanks to momentum in research. And she is now on the cusp of what was once an impossible-to-imagine adulthood.

"I keep reminding myself to calm down," she says. "You've got time."

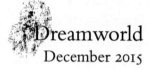

Dreamworld

December 2015

D uring the first week of the last month of 2015, as part of my job with AATB, I attended the International Summit on Human Gene Editing in Washington, DC.

Jointly hosted by the National Academy of Sciences and the National Academy of Medicine's Human Gene-Editing Initiative—alongside the Chinese Academy of Sciences and the U.K. Royal Society—the meetings brought together experts from all over the globe to talk about the many issues surrounding research that's currently being conducted to alter human genes.

Specifically, the discussion centered on a revolutionary new gene-editing technique called CRISPR, which stands for "clustered regularly interspaced short palindromic repeats." These short DNA sequences are a key component in the immune systems of bacteria.

"When viruses attack bacteria, the bacteria mobilize CRISPRs to neutralize the attack by destroying specific DNA sequences in the invading virus," said biochemist Sam Sternberg, Ph.D., who studied in one of the labs credited with making the discovery, the Doudna Lab at U.C. Berkeley, and is the author of an upcoming book about CRISPR's discovery. "By transplanting CRISPR into other kinds of cells, though, scientists have developed a new way to alter the genome."

The technique makes it possible to make specific changes in DNA—in plants, animals, and, yes, humans. Harnessed by science, CRISPR could change everything we know about medicine. CRISPR was named "2015 Breakthrough of the Year" by the American Association for the Advancement of Science, and key players in the discovery of CRISPR were nominated for the 2015 Nobel Prize for Chemistry.

Since CRISPR is so powerful and so accessible, scientists from all over the world agreed to meet to establish some ground rules for how it should be used.

This particular conference was considered the descendant of a 1975 meeting called the International Congress on Recombinant DNA Molecules, which was held at the Asilomar Conference Center in Pacific Grove, California. In 1975, biochemists and geneticists and ethicists argued about whether research into manipulating DNA was a good idea.

The concern in 1975 arose from work that Paul Berg, a renowned biochemist at Stanford and one of the meeting's organizers, was doing with simian virus 40, which could be made to cause cancer in rodents. Some scientists worried that the bacteria might escape and cause cancer in people. The meetings ended with an agreement that scientific inquiry could continue, but with restrictions to limit "unforeseen and damaging consequences for human health and Earth's ecosystems," as Berg wrote many years later in an opinion piece in the journal *Nature* called "Meetings That Changed the World."

Today, it's gene editing that's become a controversial subject. Gene editing is exciting because it has the potential to cure fatal genetic disease. Normally, a development like this would be celebrated, since it could hold the answer to many patients' prayers and stop suffering. However, gene editing might also be used for less noble purposes, which is where the controversy comes in.

A month before the summit, doctors were able to cure a little girl with previously incurable leukemia "by removing immune cells, editing them so they'd go after cancer cells while also resisting a chemotherapy drug, and then injecting them back into her," as Ed Yong wrote in the *Atlantic*. Elsewhere, researchers are working on taking cells from HIV sufferers, "deleting a gene the virus needs to stage its invasions," and putting the cells back inside the patient. This kind of application of the technology is called somatic cell therapy; it changes cells inside a person's body, and that's as far as it goes.

Many new medical advancements are met, at first, with fear. In the 1970s, along with Berg's simian virus 40, in vitro fertilization, a.k.a. the making of "test-tube babies," was perceived by some as a threat to the fabric of our society. Cloning faced the same fears in later years; stem-cell research, the same. Some experts fear that gene-editing technology will to lead to eugenics, or to breeding humans to have specific characteristics. CRISPR could be used to edit the human germ line (i.e., genes inside eggs, sperm, or embryos). If genes are changed at this level, those alterations can be inherited by future generations. Maybe that sounds ominous, but what if it's harnessed in a good way—say, to get rid of deadly and debilitating genetic diseases like Tay-Sachs and Huntington's forever?

Panelist Hille Haker, the Richard McCormick, S.J., Chair of Moral Theology at Loyola University Chicago, recommended a two-year ban on basic genetic-editing research while the experts figure out "if we should" be doing this. She also recommended that the scientific community hold off on using CRISPR to find cures for disease for those two years, arguing that we need to consider the freedom of choice of the embryo.

When I heard her comments I thought, *Freedom to have cystic fibrosis? To suffer and die as a child?* The unspoken point seemed to be: if you have a disease, it's because God wants you to have one. Patient voices were noticeably absent from the agenda.

For example, nobody was asking Jeff Carroll, an assistant professor in the Department of Psychology at Western Washington University, whose lab is looking at symptoms of Huntington's disease, what he thought. It's a subject close to his heart, since Jeff inherited the mutation. The thirty-eight-year-old knows that sometime in the next couple of decades, he'll "lose control over his body and slowly go mad, just like his mother did," wrote Antonio Regalado in the *MIT Technology Review* when he wrote about the conference.

During the Q & A, the organizers had put microphones in the audience, and I couldn't help myself—my blood was boiling from listening to all this speculation and theorizing in the face of suffering—so I decided to speak.

"I'm the mother of a child who died because of a fatal birth defect. He was six days old and he suffered every day. The look on his face was like, 'Mom, what's going on?' He had seizures every day. We donated his body for research. If you have the skills and the knowledge to fix these diseases, then freaking do it! That's it." And with that, I sat down.

NPR called me the next day to ask if I said "fricking," "frigging," or "freaking."

What Is the Answer?

Most of the people on the organ-transplant waiting list are there because of a disease—a disease that could have an alternative treatment, or even a cure. Giving a kidney to a researcher could extend the already years-long waiting list, but how much longer does the list grow if researchers cannot access the organs, eyes, or tissues they need in order to find a cure?

My dream is not to make all organ-procurement organizations and eye banks go bankrupt by recovering tissue for research. The system is set up to provide organs, eyes, and tissue for patients who need a transplant. Supplying these donations for researchers is an afterthought: many OPOs refer to these donations as "research-only," as if this were some kind of second-place or consolation prize. But the researchers may need these tissues to find a treatment or a cure for the very diseases that put those patients on the transplant waiting list. In most cases, OPOs have a monopoly on recovering organs, and they can choose not to recover an organ for research. In many organizations, this would be seen as a sound financial decision. OPO leadership might report that they cannot afford to recover organs or tissue for "research-only" donations. What can be done to change this? Researchers need tissue to conduct life-saving research, and in some cases they cannot get it, or they have to wait years.

Perhaps the processing fees for both transplant and research could be exactly the same, taking away the incentive to recover for transplant only. Perhaps this might lead to better treatments and cures, and the transplant list might decrease naturally because of this.

My Dreamworld

My dreamworld: A step toward a cure for deadly diseases like retinoblastoma, urea cycle disorder, cystic fibrosis, and anencephaly. A new treatment for cervical cancer. A medical device that can save the sickest and smallest patients through innovative intraosseous access. Training for paramedics to find an infant's airway. Cornea studies that may help restore lost vision.

Like millions of others before them, these discoveries were made possible through organ, eye, tissue, blood, and whole-body donations. In many cases, the decision to donate was made by grieving families on the worst day of their lives. Why shouldn't they ultimately know the impact of these donations? I wanted to know, and now I want to help others find answers that may give them meaning and peace, as my journey in learning about Thomas's donations did for me and my family.

Fortunately, things are changing. The National Disease Research Interchange is in the early stages of launching a program to keep donor families informed about research that involves their loved ones' donations.

In addition, OPOs across the country are learning more about neonatal donation, communicating with one another, and developing new processes. The OPO in Dallas, Southwest Transplant Alliance (STA), performed their very first neonatal donations for research in 2015, per the request of Michelle Seyl, mom of baby Alex, who was born with trisomy 18. Trisomy 18, also known as Edwards syndrome, is caused by an extra chromosome and is life-threatening. Michelle told me that because of the Philly.com story, she reached out to STA to facilitate research donations of her son's body: his brain went to the Brain Endowment Bank at the Miller School of Medicine for the study of trisomy 18 and other neurodevelopmental disorders; and his lungs went to the International Institute for the Advancement of Medicine, which matched the donation with a request from researchers investigating new treatments for cystic fibrosis.

Eversight, one of the largest consortium eye banks in the United States, has launched a donor family–researcher program to help donor families and researchers meet. This is how Eversight describes its work: "Through research, we seek to have a maximum impact on finding new cures and better therapies for those with blindness and vision loss—giving hope to millions. This program would offer a previously untapped potential and fulfill a new mission of Eversight; to provide a greater source of healing and pride for families experiencing loss. We not only help to restore and preserve sight, but we offer families hope through eye donation as an opportunity to allow their loved ones a lasting legacy. The researcher would greatly benefit from gaining a deeper understanding of the gift that makes their efforts possible. Our program would shed light on the inseparable bond between donation and finding the next cure."

In my dream world, there would be an established process for a donor's family to be more informed, if they want to be, about the research projects to which their loved one contributed. The donor's family would have the right to be notified if a study is published; they would be invited to attend events, tour facilities, and correspond with the researchers. Organ, eye, and tissue donors would be recognized with a memorial plaque in every lobby. This would go both ways: researchers would be invited to write a letter to the donor's family about their research, and they could meet if they want to. Researchers and organizations would be accustomed to this kind of interaction—the same way medical schools are now inviting donor families to deceased-donor recognition ceremonies. Alex Solomon, a student at Georgetown Medical School, explained that students there are told before the beginning of the full-

year anatomy lab that the deceased donors they will be working with will be "the most valuable teachers we'll ever have
in our medical career," and that students are expected to treat
them with the utmost respect. At the end of the course, eight
months later, the students create and conduct a remembrance
ceremony complete with readings and songs for the families
of the donors, which is held in the school's largest auditorium.
Students, faculty, and extended family are then invited to min-
gle—an invaluable opportunity for the students to thank the
donor families for their loved one's final gift.

If you are a researcher or work in an organ-procurement
organization and are approached by a family, as I approached
the facilities that received my son's gifts, here's why you don't
need to worry about this: it's completely legal within the
parameters of HIPAA and may even improve the experience of
your employees and researchers, as well as bring comfort to the
donor family. (Also, in my experience, PR teams are glad for the
opportunity to tell a positive story about what their organization does.)

In July 2013, Bethany and Eric Conkel founded Purposeful
Gift after having lost their son, Amalya, the previous year. This
is how they describe their effort: "The goal of Purposeful Gift
is to make the donation process easier for families in the future
by offering accurate information in regards to various types of
donation, as well as providing resources and support to families as they walk through their journey." Purposeful Gift has
helped parents around the world learn about research donation
options, and helps educate OPOs around the country. Thanks
to Purposeful Gift, multiple OPOs have completed their very
first neonatal research donation.

Further, the Conkels' journey with Amalya was the catalyst
for the International Institute for the Advancement of Medicine

to develop a new neonatal donor program; since Amalya's initial donation, the program has helped forty-seven other families donate to research as of this writing. Many of those were research donors, and would not have otherwise been able to donate.

Donor families are also learning more about what happens after a loved one's body is donated to a medical school to be studied by medical students. In an article in the *Atlantic* in July 2015, journalist John Tyler Allen addressed the issue of empathy for deceased donors. Dr. Jerry Vannatta, the former executive dean of the University of Oklahoma College of Medicine, introduced the idea of the Donor Luncheon, at which the families of the deceased donors who were to be studied sat down with the medical students who would be doing the studying. In the past, some medical students have coped with the unusual stress of studying a dead body by referring to the body by a nickname related to the disease the donor had or to a physical characteristic. It is Dr. Vannatta's opinion, and mine, that this is not productive for a medical student. Students need to learn not only anatomy and medical techniques, but also a kindly bedside manner and empathy. A doctor may meet a patient's family in real life, too, so it is highly relevant training to meet the family of what are often referred to as the medical students' "first patients." I would venture to say that it might even be *less* stressful for the student to meet a family of this kind, because the student was not at all involved in the diagnosis or treatment of the deceased, or in any way connected with the reason why the person died.

"The Donor Luncheon," Dr. Vannatta said, "provides a chance to close that gap, and to make it crystal-clear in [students'] minds that this was a person who lived a life—was a father, was an uncle, was an aunt, was a grandmother, was an engineer, was an architect."

As these changes take place, members of the public who don't have any point of reference in the world of medical science will start hearing about these personal stories. These positive interactions can help establish credibility, trust, and awareness in the community. This openness and transparency may lead to more confidence in making a donation for research. This awareness can help the public realize that donation to transplant isn't the only option.

My intention is not necessarily to persuade people to donate, but to compel them to make a thoughtful decision— whatever that may be. If donation is not right for you, for whatever reason, then don't do it. But if this story resonated with you, and you found yourself relating to this journey, then I recommend it. It's a decision I will be forever proud of.

My son Thomas Ethan Gray donated his eyes, liver, and cord blood to medical research; in his short but treasured life, he contributed to the advancement of modern medicine.

I only hope my life can be as relevant.

ABBREVIATIONS AND ACRONYMS

AATB	American Association of Tissue Banks
AOPO	Association of Organ Procurement Organizations
CF	cystic fibrosis
DLA	Donate Life America
ESRD	end-stage renal disease
GTEx	genotype-tissue expression
HIPAA	Health Insurance Portability and Accountability Act
IIAM	International Institute for the Advancement of Medicine
IRB	institutional review board
NAS	National Academy of Sciences
NCI	National Cancer Institute
NDRI	National Disease Research Interchange
NIH	National Institutes of Health
NISH	National Industries for the Severely Handicapped
ODEF	Old Dominion Eye Foundation
OPO	organ-procurement organization
UNOS	United Network for Organ Sharing
USCIS	U.S. Citizenship and Immigration Services
WRTC	Washington Regional Transplant Community

RESOURCES

For Donor Families Who Would Like More Information

If you would like to find out about the impact of your loved one's donation, don't be shy. Call the organization that arranged the donation (most have a Donor Family Services department; ask to speak with them), and explain that you would like more information. This happens all the time. Provide as many details and records as you can. If you like, ask them how you might be able to write a letter or even meet your loved one's recipients. In the United States, organ, eye, tissue, and blood donations are tracked in case there is ever an FDA recall due to infectious disease.

For Human-Tissue Researchers Who Would Like to Thank the Donor's Family

If you are a human-tissue researcher and you wonder about the donor or the donor's family, write them a letter or an email. Tell the donor's family what you are learning from the tissue, and invite the family to visit the lab if you like. Give your letter to the organization that provided the tissue, and ask them to deliver it to the donor's family.

For Organ, Eye, or Tissue Recipients Who Would Like to Thank Their Donors

If you are the recipient of an organ, eye, or tissue donation and wish to connect with your donor's family, contact your doctor or review your medical records to determine which organization provided the donation. Look for a donor ID number. Contact the organization that provided the tissue, provide as many details and records as you can, and let them know that you'd like to write a letter to your donor's family.

Donations for Research, Training, and Education

If you or someone you know is interested in learning more about making an organ, eye, tissue, or whole-body donation, whether diseased or healthy, or for transplant, education, training, or research, you can consult the following list of organizations that may be able to help.

National Disease Research Interchange (NDRI)
8 Penn Center, 15th Floor
1628 JFK Boulevard
Philadelphia, PA 19103
Phone: (800) 222-NDRI (6374)
www.ndriresource.org/

Register to be a donor: http://ndriresource.org/Donor-Programs/
The-Power-to-Make-A-Difference/Register-to-Donate/145/

International Institute for the Advancement of Medicine (IIAM)
125 May Street
Edison, NJ 08837
24-hour service: (800) 486-IIAM
www.iiam.org

Non-Transplant Anatomical Donation

A search is available here: www.aatb.org/Accredited-Bank-Search
Search for "Non-Transplant Anatomical Material" under "Tissue."

Transplant Donation

If you live in the United States, and would like to learn more about organ, eye, and tissue donation and register your decision to be a donor, please visit DonateLife.net.

If you do not live in the United States, you can check the following website to see if your country has a registry:

> International Registry in Organ Donation and Transplantation http://www.irodat.org/?p=database

In addition to registering online, it is a good idea to tell your family your wishes and leave them in writing in an advance directive along with your will and health-care proxy.

You can also designate your status as an organ donor on Facebook by following these instructions:

1. Click **Life Event** at the top of your Timeline.
2. Select **Health & Wellness.**
3. Select **Organ Donor.**
4. Select your audience, and then click **Save.**

Donate Life America
701 East Byrd Street, 16th Floor
Richmond, VA 23219
Phone: (804) 377-3580
http://donatelife.net/

Eye Bank Association of America
1015 18th Street NW, Suite 1010
Washington, DC 20036
Phone: (202) 775-4999
Fax: (202) 429-6036
www.restoresight.org

Organ-Procurement Organizations (OPOs) by State

For the most up-to-date information, see the Association of Organ Procurement Organizations website:

http://www.aopo.org/find-your-opo/

ALABAMA

Alabama Organ Center
502 20th Street South, Suite 502
Birmingham, AL 35233
Phone: (205) 731-9200
Fax: (205) 731-6279
www.alabamaorgancenter.org

ALASKA

LifeCenter Northwest
3650 131st Ave SE, Suite 200
Bellevue, WA 98006
Phone: (425) 201-6563
Fax: (425) 688-7641
www.lcnw.org

ARIZONA

Donor Network of Arizona
201 West Coolidge
Phoenix, AZ 85013
Phone: (602) 222-2200
Fax: (602) 222-2202
www.dnaz.org

ARKANSAS

Arkansas Regional Organ Recovery Agency
1701 Aldersgate Road, Suite 4
Little Rock, AR 72205
Phone: (501) 907-9150
Fax: (501) 372-6279
www.arora.org

Mid-America Transplant
1110 Highlands Plaza Drive East
St. Louis, MO 63110
Phone: (314) 735-8200
Fax: (314) 991-2805
www.midamericatransplant.org

Mid-South Transplant Foundation, Inc.
8001 Centerview Parkway, Suite 302
Memphis, TN 38018
Phone: (901) 328-4438
Fax: (901) 328-4462
www.midsouthtransplant.org

Southwest Transplant Alliance
5489 Blair Road
Dallas, TX 75231
Phone: (214) 522-0255
Fax: (214) 522-0430
www.organ.org

CALIFORNIA

Donor Network West
12667 Alcosta Boulevard #500
San Ramon, CA 94583
Phone: (888) 570-9400
Fax: (925) 480-3843
www.donornetworkwest.org

Sierra Donor Services
1760 Creekside Oaks Drive, Suite 220
Sacramento, CA 95833
Phone: (916) 567-1600
Fax: (916) 567-8300
www.sierradonor.org/

LifeSharing—A Donate Life Organization
3465 Camino Del Rio South, Suite 410
San Diego, CA 92108
Phone: (619) 521-1983
Fax: (619) 521-2833
www.lifesharing.org/

OneLegacy
221 South Figueroa Street, Suite 500
Los Angeles, CA 90012
Phone: (213) 229-5600
Fax: (213) 229-5601
www.onelegacy.org

COLORADO
Donor Alliance
720 South Colorado Boulevard, Suite 800-N
Denver, CO 80246
Phone: (303) 329-4747
Fax: (303) 321-1183
www.donoralliance.org

CONNECTICUT
New England Organ Bank
60 First Avenue
Waltham, MA 02451
Phone: (617) 244-8000
Fax: (617) 244-8755
www.neob.org

LifeChoice Donor Services
340 West Newberry Road, Suite A
Bloomfield, CT 06002
Phone: (860) 545-4143
Fax: (800) 874-5215
www.lifechoiceopo.org

DELAWARE
Gift of Life Donor Program
401 North 3rd Street
Philadelphia, PA 19123
Phone: (215) 557-8090
Fax: (215) 557-9359
www.donors1.org

DISTRICT OF COLUMBIA
Washington Regional Transplant Community
7619 Little River Turnpike, Suite 900
Annandale, VA 22002
Phone: (703) 641-0100
Fax: (703) 658-0711
www.beadonor.org

FLORIDA
LifeQuest Organ Recovery Services
Ayers Medical Plaza, North Tower
720 SW 2nd Avenue, Suite 570
Gainesville, FL 32610
Phone: (352) 733-0350
Fax: (352) 733–0353
www.lifequestfla.org

Life Alliance Organ Recovery Agency
225 NE 34 Street, Suite 100
Miami, FL 33137
Phone: (305) 243-7622
Fax: (305) 243-7628
www.surgery.med.miami.edu/laora

TransLife
1560 Orange Avenue, Suite 400
Winter Park, FL 32789
Phone: (407) 644-3770

Fax: (407) 644-8876
www.translife.org/

LifeLink of Florida
409 Bayshore Boulevard
Tampa, FL 33606
Phone: (813) 348-6308
Fax: (813) 349-6515
www.lifelinkfoundation.org

GEORGIA
LifeLink of Georgia
2875 Northwoods Parkway
Norcross, GA 30071
Phone: (770) 225-5465
Fax: (770) 255-5454
www.lifelinkfoundation.org

Tennessee Donor Services
1600 Hayes Street, Suite 300
Nashville, TN 37203
Phone: (865) 588-1031
Fax: (865) 588-5903
www.dcids.org

HAWAII
Legacy of Life Hawai'i
405 North Kuakini Street, Suite 800
Honolulu, HI 96817
Phone: (808) 599-7630
Fax: (808) 599-7631
www.legacyoflifehawaii.org

IDAHO
Pacific Northwest Transplant Bank
2611 SW 3rd Avenue, Suite 320

Portland, OR 97201
Phone: (503) 494-5560
Fax: (503) 494-4725
www.pntb.org

Intermountain Donor Services
230 South 500 East, Suite 290
Salt Lake City, UT 84102
Phone: (801) 521-1755
Fax: (801) 364-8815
www.idslife.org

LifeCenter Northwest
3650 131st Avenue SE, Suite 200
Bellevue, WA 98006
Phone: (425) 201-6563
Fax: (425) 688-7641
www.lcnw.org

ILLINOIS
Gift of Hope Organ & Tissue Donor Network
425 Spring Lake Drive
Itasca, IL 60143
Phone: (630) 758-2600
Fax: (630) 758-2716
www.giftofhope.org

Mid-America Transplant
1110 Highlands Plaza Drive East
St. Louis, MO 63110
Phone: (314) 735-8200
Fax: (314) 991-2805
www.midamericatransplant.org

UW Organ and Tissue Donation
450 Science Drive, Suite 220

Madison, WI 53711
Phone: (608) 262-3248
Fax: (608) 262-9099
www.uwhealth.org/organ-donation/organ-and-tissue-donation/10868

INDIANA
Indiana Donor Network
3760 Guion Road
Indianapolis, IN 46222
Phone: (317) 685-0389
Fax: (317) 685-1687
www.indianadonornetwork.org

Kentucky Organ Donor Affiliates
10160 Linn Station Road
Louisville, KY 40223
Phone: (502) 581-9511
Fax: (502) 589-5157
www.kyorgandonor.org

LifeCenter Organ Donor Network
615 Elsinore Place, Suite 400
Cincinnati, OH 45202
Phone: (513) 558-8997
Fax: (513) 558-8843
www.lifepassiton.org

Gift of Hope Organ & Tissue Donor Network
425 Spring Lake Drive
Itasca, IL 60143
Phone: (630) 758-2600
Fax: (630) 758-2716
www.giftofhope.org

IOWA
Iowa Donor Network
550 Madison Avenue

North Liberty, IA 52317
Phone: (319) 665-3787
Fax: (319) 665-3788
www.iowadonornetwork.org

Nebraska Organ Recovery System
8502 West Center Road
Omaha, NE 68124
Phone: (402) 733-1800
Fax: (402) 733-9312
http://www.nedonation.org/

KANSAS
Midwest Transplant Network
1900 W 47th Place, Suite 400
Westwood, KS 66205
Phone: (913) 262-1668
Fax: (913) 262-5130
www.mwtn.org

KENTUCKY
Kentucky Organ Donor Affiliates
10160 Linn Station Road
Louisville, KY 40223
Phone: (502) 581-9511
Fax: (502) 589-5157
www.kyorgandonor.org

LifeCenter Organ Donor Network
615 Elsinore Place, Suite 400
Cincinnati, OH 45202
Phone: (513) 558-5000
Fax: (513) 558-8843
www.lifepassiton.org

Tennessee Donor Services
1600 Hayes Street, Suite 300

Nashville, TN 37203
Phone: (865) 588-1031
Fax: (865) 588-5903
tds.dcids.org

LOUISIANA

The Louisiana Organ Procurement Agency
4441 North I-10 Service Road
Metairie, LA 70002
Phone: (504) 837-3355
Fax: (504) 833-7894
www.lopa.org

MAINE

New England Organ Bank
60 First Avenue
Waltham, MA 02451
Phone: (617) 244-8000
Fax: (617) 244-8755
www.neob.org

MARYLAND

The Living Legacy Foundation of Maryland
1730 Twin Springs Road, Suite 200
Baltimore, MD 21227
Phone: (410) 242-7000
Fax: (410) 242-1871
www.thellf.org

Washington Regional Transplant Community
7619 Little River Turnpike, Suite 900
Annandale, VA 22002
Phone: (703) 641-0100
Fax: (703) 658-0711
www.beadonor.org

MASSACHUSETTS
New England Organ Bank
60 First Avenue
Waltham, MA 02451
Phone: (617) 244-8000
Fax: (617) 244-8755
www.neob.org

LifeChoice Donor Services
340 West Newberry Road, Suite A
Bloomfield, CT 06002
Phone: (800) 874-5215
Fax: (860) 545-4143
www.lifechoiceopo.org

MICHIGAN
Gift of Life Michigan
3861 Research Park Drive
Ann Arbor, MI 48108
Phone: (734) 973-1577
Fax: (734) 973-3133
www.giftoflifemichigan.org

UW Organ and Tissue Donation
450 Science Drive, Suite 220
Madison, WI 53711
Phone: (608) 262-3248
Fax: (608) 262-9099
www.uwhealth.org/organ-donation/organ-and-tissue-donation/10868

MINNESOTA
LifeSource Organ and Tissue Donation
2225 West River Road North
Minneapolis, MN 55411
Phone: (612) 800-6100

Fax: (612) 800-6331
www.life-source.org

UW Organ and Tissue Donation
450 Science Drive, Suite 220
Madison, WI 53711
Phone: (608) 262-3248
Fax: (608) 262-9099
www.uwhealth.org/organ-donation/organ-and-tissue-
donation/10868

Mississippi Organ Recovery Agency
4400 Lakeland Drive
Flowood, MS 39232
Phone: (601) 933-1000
Fax: (601) 933-1006
www.msora.org

Mid-South Transplant Foundation, Inc.
8001 Centerview Parkway, Suite 302
Memphis, TN 38018
Phone: (901) 328-4438
Fax: (901) 328-4462
www.midsouthtransplant.org

Midwest Transplant Network
1900 W 47th Place, Suite 400
Westwood, KS 66205
Phone: (913) 262-1668
Fax: (913) 262-5130
www.mwtn.org

Mid-America Transplant
1110 Highlands Plaza Drive East

St. Louis, MO 63110
Phone: (314) 735-8200
Fax: (314) 991-2805
www.midamericatransplant.org

MONTANA
LifeCenter Northwest
3650 131st Ave SE, Suite 200
Bellevue, WA 98006
Phone: (425) 201-6563
Fax: (425) 688-7641
www.lcnw.org

NEBRASKA
Nebraska Organ Recovery System
8502 West Center Road
Omaha, NE 68124
Phone: (402) 733-1800
Fax: (402) 733-9312
www.nedonation.org

Iowa Donor Network
550 Madison Avenue
North Liberty, IA 52317
Phone: (319) 665-3787
Fax: (319) 665-3788
www.iowadonornetwork.org

NEVADA
Nevada Donor Network
2061 East Sahara Avenue
Las Vegas, NV 89104
Phone: (702) 796-9600
Fax: (702) 796-4225
www.nvdonor.org

Intermountain Donor Services
230 South 500 East, Suite 290
Salt Lake City, UT 84102
Phone: (801) 521-1755
Fax: (801) 364-8815
www.idslife.org

Donor Network West
12667 Alcosta Boulevard #500
San Ramon, CA 94583
Phone: (888) 570-9400
Fax: (510) 444-8501
www.donornetworkwest.org

NEW HAMPSHIRE
New England Organ Bank
60 First Avenue
Waltham, MA 02451
Phone: (617) 244-8000
Fax: (617) 244-8755
www.neob.org

NEW JERSEY
Gift of Life Donor Program
401 North 3rd Street
Philadelphia, PA 19123
Phone: (215) 557-8090
Fax: (215) 557-9359
www.donors1.org

NJ Sharing Network
691 Central Avenue
New Providence, NJ 07974
Phone: (908) 516-5400
Fax: (908) 516-5501
www.njsharingnetwork.org

NEW MEXICO
New Mexico Donor Services
1609 University Boulevard NE
Albuquerque, NM 87102
Phone: (505) 843-7672
Fax: (505) 343-1828
www.donatelifenm.org

NEW YORK
Center for Donation & Transplant
Albany Medical Center
218 Great Oaks Boulevard
Albany, NY 12203
Phone: (518) 262-5606
Fax: (518) 262-5427
www.cdtny.org

Unyts
110 Broadway
Buffalo, NY 14203
Phone: (716) 853-6667
Fax: (716) 853-6674
www.unyts.org

LiveOnNY
460 West 34th Street, 15th Floor
New York, NY 10001
Phone: (646) 291-4444
Fax: (646) 291-4600
www.liveonny.org

Finger Lakes Donor Recovery Network
Corporate Woods Brighton, Building 30, Suite 220
Rochester, NY 14623
Phone: (585) 272-4930
Fax: (585) 272-4956
www.donorrecovery.org

Center for Organ Recovery & Education
RIDC Park
204 Sigma Drive
Pittsburgh, PA 15238
Phone: (412) 963-3550
Fax: (412) 963-3564
www.core.org

NORTH CAROLINA

Carolina Donor Services
909 East Arlington Boulevard
Greenville, NC 27858
Phone: (252) 757-0090
Fax: (252) 757-0708
www.carolinadonorservices.org

LifeShare of the Carolinas
5000 D Airport Center Parkway
Charlotte, NC 28208
Phone: (704) 512-3303
Fax: (704) 512-3056
www.lifesharecarolinas.org

LifeNet Health
1864 Concert Drive
Virginia Beach, VA 23453
Phone: (800) 847-7831
Fax: (757) 227-4690
www.lifenethealth.org

NORTH DAKOTA

LifeSource Organ and Tissue Donation
2225 West River Road North
Minneapolis, MN 55411
Phone: (612) 800-6100
Fax: (612) 800-6331
www.life-source.org

OHIO

LifeCenter Organ Donor Network
615 Elsinore Place, Suite 400
Cincinnati, OH 45202
Phone: (513) 558-5000
Fax: (513) 558-8843
www.lifepassiton.org

Life Connection of Ohio
3661 Briarfield Boulevard #105
Maumee, OH 43537-1694
Phone: (419) 893-4891
Fax: (419) 893-1827
www.lifeconnectionofohio.org

Lifebanc
4775 Richmond Road
Cleveland, OH 44128-5919
Phone: (216) 752-5433
Fax: (216) 751-4204
www.lifebanc.org

Lifeline of Ohio
770 Kinnear Road, Suite 200
Columbus, OH 43212
Phone: (614) 291-5667
Fax: (614) 291-0660
www.lifelineofohio.org

Kentucky Organ Donor Affiliates
10160 Linn Station Road
Louisville, KY 40223
Phone: (502) 581-9511
Fax: (502) 589-5157
www.kyorgandonor.org

OKLAHOMA
LifeShare Transplant Donor Services of Oklahoma
4705 NW Expressway
Oklahoma City, OK 73132
Phone: (405) 840-5551
Fax: (405) 840-9748
www.lifeshareoklahoma.org

OREGON
Pacific Northwest Transplant Bank
2611 SW 3rd Avenue, Suite 320
Portland, OR 97201
Phone: (503) 494-5560
Fax: (503) 494-4725
www.pntb.org

PENNSYLVANIA
Gift of Life Donor Program
401 North 3rd Street
Philadelphia, PA 19123
Phone: (215) 557-8090
Fax: (215) 557-9359
www.donors1.org

Center for Organ Recovery & Education
RIDC Park, 204 Sigma Drive
Pittsburgh, PA 15238
Phone: (412) 963-3550
Fax: (412) 963-3564
www.core.org

LiveOnNY
460 West 34th Street, 15th Floor
New York, NY 10001
Phone: (646) 291-4444
Fax: (646) 291-4600
www.liveonny.org

PUERTO RICO
LifeLink of Puerto Rico
Daimler-Chrysler Building, Metro Office Park
Suite 100, Calle 1, #1
Guaynabo, PR 00968-1705
Phone: (787) 277-0300
Fax: (787) 277-0876
www.lifelinkfoundation.org

RHODE ISLAND
New England Organ Bank
60 First Avenue
Waltham, MA 02451
Phone: (617) 244-8000
Fax: (617) 244-8755
www.neob.org

SOUTH CAROLINA
LifePoint
3950 Faber Place Drive
Charleston, SC 29405
Phone: (843) 763–7755
Fax: (843) 763–6393
www.lifepoint-sc.org

LifeLink of Georgia
2875 Northwoods Parkway
Norcross, GA 30071
(770) 225-5465
(800) 544-6667
www.lifelinkfoundation.org

SOUTH DAKOTA
LifeSource Organ and Tissue Donation
2225 West River Road North
Minneapolis, MN 55411
Phone: (612) 800-6100

Fax: (612) 800–63311
www.life-source.org

Tennessee Donor Services
1600 Hayes Street, Suite 300
Nashville, TN 37203
Phone: (865) 588-1031
Fax: (865) 588-5903
tds.dcids.org

Mid-South Transplant Foundation, Inc.
8001 Centerview Parkway, Suite 302
Memphis, TN 38018
Phone: (901) 328-4438
Fax: (901) 328-4462
www.midsouthtransplant.org

LifeGift
2510 Westridge Street
Houston, TX 77054
Phone: (713) 523-4438
Fax: (713) 737-8110
www.lifegift.org

Southwest Transplant Alliance
5489 Blair Road
Dallas, TX 75231
Phone: (214) 522-0255
Fax: (214) 522-0430
www.organ.org

Texas Organ Sharing Alliance
8122 Datapoint Drive, Suite 200
San Antonio, TX 78229

Phone: (210) 614-7030
Fax: (210) 614-2129
www.txorgansharing.org

UTAH

Intermountain Donor Services
230 South 500 East, Suite 290
Salt Lake City, UT 84102
Phone: (801) 521-1755
Fax: (801) 364-8815
www.idslife.org

VERMONT

Center for Donation & Transplant
Albany Medical Center
218 Great Oaks Boulevard
Albany, NY 12203
Phone: (518) 262-5606
Fax: (518) 262-5427
www.cdtny.org

New England Organ Bank
60 First Avenue
Waltham, MA 02451
Phone: (617) 244-8000
Fax: (617) 244-8755
www.neob.org

VIRGINIA

LifeNet Health
1864 Concert Drive
Virginia Beach, VA 23453
Phone: (800) 847-7831
Fax: (757) 227-4690
www.lifenethealth.org

Washington Regional Transplant Community
7619 Little River Turnpike, Suite 900
Annandale, VA 22002
Phone: (703) 641-0100
Fax: (703) 658-0711
www.beadonor.org

Tennessee Donor Services
1600 Hayes Street, Suite 300
Nashville, TN 37203
Phone: (865) 588-1031
Fax: (865) 588-5903
tds.dcids.org

Carolina Donor Services
909 East Arlington Boulevard
Greenville, NC 27858
Phone: (252) 757-0090
Fax: (252) 757-0708
www.carolinadonorservices.org

WASHINGTON

LifeCenter Northwest
3650 131st Avenue SE, Suite 200
Bellevue, WA 98006
Phone: (425) 201-6563
Fax: (425) 688-7641
www.lcnw.org

Pacific Northwest Transplant Bank
2611 SW 3rd Avenue, Suite 320
Portland, OR 97201
Phone: (503) 494-5560
Fax: (503) 494-4725
www.pntb.org

WEST VIRGINIA

Center for Organ Recovery & Education
RIDC Park, 204 Sigma Drive
Pittsburgh, PA 15238
Phone: (412) 963-3550
Fax: (412) 963-3564
www.core.org

Kentucky Organ Donor Affiliates
10160 Linn Station Road
Louisville, KY 40223
Phone: (502) 581-9511
Fax: (502) 589-5157
www.kyorgandonor.org

LifeLine of Ohio
770 Kinnear Road, Suite 200
Columbus, OH 43212
Phone: (614) 291-5667
Fax: (614) 291-0660
www.lifelineofohio.org

LifeNet Health
1864 Concert Drive
Virginia Beach, VA 23453
Phone: (800) 847-7831
Fax: (757) 227-4690
www.lifenethealth.org

WISCONSIN

UW Organ and Tissue Donation
450 Science Drive, Suite 220
Madison, WI 53711
Phone: (608) 262-3248
Fax: (608) 262-9099
www.uwhealth.org/organ-donation/organ-and-tissue-donation/10868

Wisconsin Donor Network
9000 West Chester Street, Suite 250
Milwaukee, WI 53214
Phone: (414) 937-6999
Fax: (414) 937-6998
www.bcw.edu/bcw/Organ-Tissue-Marrow/index.htm

LifeSource Organ and Tissue Donation
2225 West River Road North
Minneapolis, MN 55411
Phone: (612) 800-6100
Fax: (612) 800-6331
www.life-source.org

WYOMING

Donor Alliance
720 South Colorado Boulevard, Suite 800-N
Denver, CO 80246
Phone: (303) 329-4747
Fax: (303) 321-1183
www.donoralliance.org

Intermountain Donor Services
230 South 500 East, Suite 290
Salt Lake City, UT 84102
Phone: (801) 521-1755
Fax: (801) 364-8815
www.idslife.org

Outside the USA
VIRGIN ISLANDS

LifeLink of Puerto Rico
Daimler-Chrysler Building, Metro Office Park
Suite 100, Calle 1, #1
Guaynabo, PR 00968-1705
Phone: (787) 277-0300
Fax: (787) 277-0876
www.lifelinkfoundation.org

ACKNOWLEDGMENTS

My sincere gratitude goes out to the following:

Those who brought this book to life through their hard work and passion: Nicole James, Rachel Sussman, and Terra Chalberg of Chalberg & Sussman; Mark James; Elizabeth Stein; Luke Dempsey, Suzanne Wickham, Kim Dayman, and Adrian Morgan at HarperOne, and Mary Ann Petyak at HarperCollins; Dan Gerstein; and Professor Joseph Graf.

The medical staff who handled our challenging situation with professionalism, kindness, and grace under pressure: John Maddox; Harvey Stern; Ahmet Baschat; Christopher Harman; Alfred Khoury; Samer Cheaib; Stephen Kennedy; Kelly Gallo; Philip Brooks; Brandy Celnicker; Becky Taylor; the team from Capital Caring, especially Cindi Carney; and Metropolitan Funeral Service, especially Karen Brendle.

The entire team at WRTC, especially Becky Hill, Lisa A. Colaianni, Maureen M. Balderston, Immanuel Rasool, Karen Haase, Debra Goldstein, Lori Brigham, Carlos Fernandez-Bueno, Elizabeth Turner, Rudy Murray, Dave Destefano, Kimberly Woodard, Connie Marroquin, and Matthew Niles.

The entire team at Old Dominion Eye Foundation, especially Bill Proctor, Christina Jenkins, Jennifer Payton, and David Taylor.

The entire team at NDRI, especially Bill Leinweber, Jeffrey Thomas, Mike Salvatore, Bernadette Mestichelli, and Kerri Harvey.

The entire team at Massachusetts Eye and Ear/Schepens Eye Research Institute, especially Elizabeth Mason, Carolyn Bellefeuille, James Zieske, Andrius Kazlauskas, Patricia D'Amore, John Fernandez, Mary Leach, and Jennifer Street.

The entire team at Duke Center for Human Genetics, especially

Heidi Cope, Simon Gregory, Allison Ashley-Koch, Deidre Krupp, and Karen Soldano.

The entire team at Cytonet, especially Mark Johnston, Sonya Meheux, and Kyle Kinsey.

The entire team at the University of Pennsylvania Genetics Lab, especially Arupa Ganguly, Karen Kreeger, Jennifer Richards-Yutz, and Jessica Ebrahimzadeh.

To those who served as invaluable sources of information, facts, ideas, and edits: Misha Angrist, the Conkel family, the McGinley and Cates families, Scotty Bolleter, Sue Scott, Christian Hinrichs, Mara ans Sharon Cray, Chris Mason, Albert Wu, Sarah Grays, Sam Sternberg, Laura Siminoff, Rebecca Cummings-Suppi, Carol Weil, Keith Meatto, Jeremy Wrubel, Veronica Fernandez, Alex Ampadu, Jackie Lue Raia, Alex Solomon, James Selby Jr., Veena Chowdhan and Abbas Syed, Anthony DiMaria, Amanda Bisnauth-Thomas, Matt Might, Sukru Emre, Michael Vitez, Ronda Horstman, Gregory Grossman, Hilary Czarda, Gina Dunne-Smith, and Jerry Vannetta.

Influences, contributors to the story, and help along the way: Houeida Saad, Monika and Anouk Jaquier and the entire Anencephaly.info Facebook Group community, Allison and Faith Andrews, Cyndi and Morgan Barnett, Tania Ponomarenko, Adam Foster, Jay and Clarice Gibson, Ozan Williams, Azian Zain, Anna Whiston-Donaldson, Sophia Smith, Emily Berman, Tony Zwerdling and Ginger Vowell, Deb Weisshaar, Min Tak, Jane Jamieson, and Caitriona Palmer.

The entire AATB staff, especially Frank Wilton, Scott Brubaker, Jenny Chatman, and Veronica Escalona.

To those who donated the blood and blood products that I received during childbirth (Inova Blood Bank Donor IDs #: W0B9810002415, W089810002346, W089810602156, W089810201081, W083210000091, W089810602001, and W089809453744), thank you for donating the blood that saved my life. I hope to meet you all and thank you in person.

My amazing family and friends who endured it all with us, especially Suzanne Rydel and the entire Hughes family, Mark and Jennifer Walpole, Ethan Walpole, James and Cathy Walpole and the entire

Walpole family, Bob Rydel[2] and family, Pauline and Eddie Gray and family, Julia and Garry Mountford, Susan Pollack, and Melanie and Chris Parks.

My children, Callum and Jocelyn. I hope you can always feel me hugging you.

And the other person who experienced this with me, my husband, Ross. I'm so glad to have you by my side.

ABOUT THE AUTHOR

Sarah Gray is an organ, eye, and tissue donation advocate and a public speaker. She is the director of communications for the American Association of Tissue Banks in McLean, Virginia. She lives in Washington, DC, with her husband, Ross, and their children, Callum and Jocelyn.